T0195010

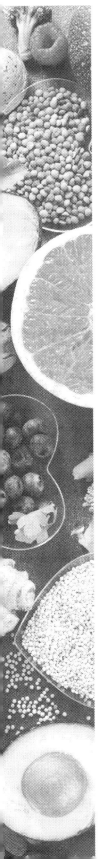

Nutrients, Vitamins, Minerals and Hydration for Health Restoration

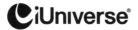

NUTRIENTS, VITAMINS, MINERAL AND HYDRATION FOR HEALTH RESTORATION

iUniverse books may be ordered through booksellers or by contacting:

iUniverse
1663 Liberty Drive
Bloomington, IN 47403
www.iuniverse.com
844-349-9409

Because of the dynamic nature of the Internet, any web addresses or links contained in this book may have changed since publication and may no longer be valid. The views expressed in this work are solely those of the author and do not necessarily reflect the views of the publisher, and the publisher hereby disclaims any responsibility for them.

Any people depicted in stock imagery provided by Getty Images are models, and such images are being used for illustrative purposes only.
Certain stock imagery © Getty Images.

You should not undertake any diet/exercise regimen recommended in this book before consulting your personal physician. Neither the author nor the publisher shall be responsible or liable for any loss or damage allegedly arising as a consequence of your use or application of any information or suggestions contained in this book.

ISBN: 978-1-6632-3740-8(sc)
ISBN: 978-1-6632-3739-2 (e)

Library of Congress Control Number: 2022905293

Print information available on the last page.

iUniverse rev. date: 09/09/2022

Contents

Acknowledgement

1. The continuous support and prayers of my children and family and friends are deeply appreciated.

2. Editor-in-Chief of iUniverse is highly appreciated for time taken to review this manuscript.

3. This book could not have attained its scholarly astute without the professional review of the Reviewers, words are not enough to express my gratitude to you all.

4. I am immensely grateful to all the consultants that contributed their skills to ensure that this book takes a professional status, I cannot thank you enough.

Dedication

This book is dedicated to all who got sick, disabled or died of preventable diseases such as highlighted in this book and to Almighty God who made this accomplishment possible.

Preface

The mission of this author since 2008 remains to contribute own quota at ensuring that community is educated about the potency and healing power of food and herbs. In that way, whether someone can afford costly modern treatment or not, the knowledge and use of healing foods, food supplements, and herbs provides an effective alternative. Since 2008 that this author launched a nutritional investigation on the connection between nutrition and health and illness, this author has published other books and academic articles along that line and social determinant of health.

This author is a Certified Health Education Specialist (CHES˚), possesses a Diploma in Nutrition and Fitness, and bachelors degree in Food Science. Also, she has Masters degree in Business Administration (MBA), Masters degree in Public Health (MPH), and Doctor of Philosophy (PhD) in Public Health with a concentration in Community Health.

This author's source of motivation was obtained from the positive outcomes and testimonies of persons who benefited from her effort. Since 2008, this author's use of health education, nutrition assessment, nutrition and herbal remedies has brought healing and restoration of health to patients. Among the most remarkable beneficiaries was a young man who sustained injury from motorcycle accident and received medical treatments for his injury for months and the wound refused to heal, and instead, the injury went progressively bad. It became swollen, moved from light to dark colour and dripped fluid that oozed out offensive odour. The leg was localized and it caused the patient to be bedridden and unbearable pain, and patient could no longer use his leg to move. Author suggested nutraceutical to him and he used it, and the injury healed and dried up in less than one week. The young man went crazy with gratitude to this author.

The second was in 2012, a lady, an American citizen who went through mammogram diagnosis twice and there were lumps in her breasts in the United States, author placed her on a three-week nutraceutical therapy and after the treatment, she went back for another mammogram and the lumps disappeared to date. Some other beneficiaries were people who suffered from hypertension, the types that were resistant to drugs with systolic reading of above 170, within three months of receiving nutritional assessment, health education, change of nutrition and use of nutraceuticals, their blood pressure went down to normal.

The author's mother also benefited, she was once obese, hypertensive, sick and frail, and could not do much to help her or do her occupation, which was farming for several years. This author assessed her nutrition and redirected her on a healthy line and using nutraceutical and healthy nutrition she lost all the weight in a space of three to six months, and became so strong that she resumed her normal life activities and did her farming in a significant manner that she boasted about her farm and how well her plants were doing because she did it herself.

The author was not left out on the list of beneficiaries, prior to 2008, this author experienced acute constipation that lingered on, author could only eat small amount of food and it took up to four hours to digest. Additionally, this author suffered from severe pains and aches inside her legs, and doctors could not find anything wrong with her legs or the author. Through the author's continuous investigation, she discovered the solutions and from 2008 to date, she never experienced any of those and she has enjoyed a generous amount of food. The list goes on and on. Author is thankful to the nature that she has no metabolic syndrome diseases presently.

This author is determined to ensure that no one lives in pain, disability or die of illnesses that are preventable. Thus, this author deemed it necessary to promote the healing power of nutrients, minerals and vitamins to the body through health education provided in this book.

The author's ideology has a connection with the ancient health restoration practice. A French biochemist by name Casmire Funk was the first to identify the need for what he called 'accessory growth factor' in human body, which he named vitamins. Also, history informs us that certain illnesses amounted from lack or deficiency of certain nutrients from the body, and some diseases arose from excessive consumption of certain nutrients. For instance, scurvy was a disease of the mouth caused by deficiency of vitamin C, rickets was caused by deficiency of vitamin D, and beriberi a disease caused by lack of vitamin B. A few more examples are, anemia caused by disorder of the digestive system, low blood and low iron. Pallegra, a disease caused by deficiency of vitamin B5, and deficiency of vitamin E caused female rats to abort pregnancies, and male to become sterile. Deficiency of vitamin B6 caused dermatitis (1, 2, 3, 4).

When the lacking nutrients that caused the diseases were consumed at optimum quantity, the diseases disappeared and health was restored. For examples, daily liver intake treated anemia. Food and animal irradiation resulted in increases in vitamin D2 that treated rickets and diseases caused by deficiency of vitamin D. Vitamin A was used to cure night blindness, and xerophthalmia caused by conjuctivitis. Liver, original and fresh palm oil, unripe plantain, egg, cheese, oily fish, carrot, green leafy vegetables, apricot, and paw paw contain vitamin A at varying levels (1, 2, 3, 4).

In proposing a theory of vitamin, a scholar by name, Funk stated that there were protective factors that natural food consist of, and that those factors were vitamins that prevented a disease called beriberi. Vitamin was derived from the words "vital, amine" Amine is a word for nitrogen. Then, Funk believed that all vitamins contain nitrogen; however, scientists later discovered that not all vitamins contain nitrogen. Thus, researchers suggested that *it is necessary to discover what vitamin that is lacking in the sick* or ill person before administering treatment (3). For example vitamin A facilitates growth in rat so, to treat stunted growth in rat, it would be good to determine the vitamin A level and other deficient nutrients and supply it to optimum level, allow some healing time, before taking other medical steps (1, 2, 3, 4). The question for us here is: **Is this practice of determining the lacking nutrient/s in the ill before administering treatment enforced yet?** We need to supply the answer. Please, note that emergency situations are different, and should treated as such.

Despite these facts, people generally seek for modern medications first whenever they are ill; not minding the huge adverse effects of modern medicine on human health for short- and long-term use. Adverse effect and the huge cost of treating chronic diseases is now prompting many to seek for alternative means of preventing and treating diseases. Nutraceutical-foods that have medicinal properties have the potency to prevent or heal diseases. They are included among food supplements in the United States.

The potency of food to prevent and heal diseases, which is actually, **nothing new but, rather simply ignored.** Influential people were blamed for the derailment of medical practice from the ancient practice of determining, which nutrient is lacking in the a patient first before medical treatment. Nutrition and herbal potency is once again experiencing a revolutionary interest by scholars, researchers, and business merchants globally. It is never too late to make an amendment!

Once more, this author maintains that a significant health restoration is achievable through the optimum consumption of macronutrients, vitamins, minerals, and water. The evidence above are scientific and native medicine theory supports the author's ideology. Human life is precious and it is wealth itself.

Introduction

In this book, we will learn about macronutrients such as water, carbohydrates, proteins, lipids, fibre and ash, as well as micronutrients namely vitamins, and minerals. The lessons were presented in chapters to make learning easy. This book focused essentially, on macronutrients, minerals and vitamins, and their functions to the body, as well as the effect of their deficiencies and excessive intake to the body. Also, treated were the food sources of macronutrients, minerals and vitamins, and the healing power of hydration. Major topics were presented in chapters one to 42 and minor topics with subheadings. The lessons focused on nutrients namely, macronutrients and micronutrients, and the classes of nutrients.

Macronutrient is a scientific word used to name food needed in the body in large amount namely, water, carbohydrates, proteins, lipids, and fibre. Micronutrients is also a scientific word used to describe vitamins, minerals, and trace elements. Vitamins are organic nutrients needed in the body to perform specific essential functions. Vitamins consist of fat-soluble vitamins namely, vitamins A D E K (ADEK), and water-soluble vitamins, which include, vitamin C, and B-group vitamins. Contrary to vitamins that are organic food substances, minerals are inorganic food substances examples, calcium, sodium, potassium, magnesium, phosphorus, iron, manganese, copper, cobalt, chlorine and others.

There were some overviews or general lessons and specific lessons about the nutrients. Each chapter provided a description about each nutrient, the functions that it performs to the body, and the effects of deficiency and excessive consumption of each nutrients to the body. Also, included were sources of nutrients, and the recommended dietary allowance of nutrients. Additionally, this author provided clarifications about myths and facts in nutrition and health, and discussed the factors that affect nutrients and mineral availability and absorption. Further, the impact of food processing on nutrients was discussed, and expert effort to provide remedies to nutrient lost to food processing, which led to biofortification and mineral fortification was discussed in this nutrition book.

In nutrition science, scholars had hard times attempting to give a universally acceptable definition to the word "essentiality" of nutrient. This author also made an attempt to define the word "essentiality". Additionally, glossary was included in the end. Now you are welcome to carefully read through the book to learn the necessary lessons; starting from chapter one.

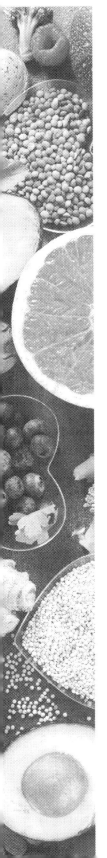

Chapter 1

Food (Macronutrients)

Food may be defined as *any substance that can be metabolized by an animal to give energy, repair and build tissue*. It may be described as *food and drink* or *anything that provides mental stimulus for thinking* (9). Food and Nutrition Board, described nutrients as chemical substances or component of food that are essential for life, tissue growth and repair. The nutrients that the body cannot produce are called essential or indispensable nutrients because, their deficiency in the body cause the body to develop diseases, prevent growth and in some cases cause death (1, 2, 3, 4, 5, 6).

Following the animal growth model, essential nutrient was described from 1960-1970 as, a deficiency of essential nutrients that prevent life cycle (growth, development, or maturation including reproduction) or cause death. Six conditions were indicated for an element to be regarded as essential. Among the condition is the sixth condition, which is that the element must cause a consistent adverse alteration of biological function from performing at optimal capacity, and such change could be prevented or reversed when the physiological quantity of the element is raised to normal or optimum (1, 2, 3, 4, 5, 6).

Currently, the most acceptable description of essential element is that it must have a definite biological function. As a result of the controversies between 1980s and 1990s over definition of essential element, there is no universally accepted list of essential elements. Food is nutrient, and nutrient may be described as that substance, which the body requires for its metabolism, growth and all body functions (7, 8). There are two major types of nutrients namely; macronutrient and micronutrient. Macro is a Greek word meaning large so; macronutrients are the nutrients that the body need in large quantities namely, carbohydrates, protein, fats and oils, and water. Micronutrients are needed by the body in small quantities namely, minerals, vitamins, and trace elements (5, 3, 6, 4).

Food is a substance, which when ingested (eaten), it is digested to separate the waste from the desired product, absorbed into the body for the body's daily needs; namely, body health, and metabolic processes namely, energy generation, growth, repair, detoxification and removal of wastes and poisonous substances out of the body and host of other biochemical reactions that take place within the body. Food can come in the form of solid, semi-solid or liquid forms (10, 5). The amount of energy or calories needed by the body to perform its function such as breathing, blood circulation, food digestion, and maintenance of the body temperature when at rest is called basal metabolic rate (BMR) (5, 9).

Basal or basic Metabolic Rate (BMR) Calculation

Harris-Benedict use age, gender, weight and height to calculate BMR for a person. Using Harris-Benedict formulae to calculate BMR for female, and male (71, 72):

Male: 66 + (13.7 x weight in kg) + (5 x height in cm)- (6.8 x age in years) = Male BMR

Female: 655+ (9.6 x weight in kg) + (1.8 x height in cm)-(4.7 x age in years) = Female BMR.

Daily Calorie Requirement for Male and Female Based Upon Physical Activities

Also, one size of BMR cannot fit all, because each person's physical activity or energy expenditure varies. To further narrow down a person's specific daily calorie requirement, there is a need to include various perspectives of a person's physical activities and energy expenditure (71, 72). For example, a person's specific daily calorie requirement will be calculated as follows: Male BMR times energy needed to perform specific activity namely, sedentary (1.2), light activity (1.375), moderate active, (1.55) very active (1.725), and extra active (1.9). The same applies to female. Specific lifestyle daily energy requirement is to be calculated this way:

For a male that sits always and do not do any physical activity or do very small activity, which is sedentary lifestyle your daily energy requirement would be calculated this way (71, 72):

Sedentary Male = Male BMR x 1.2.

If you are a female with the same sedentary lifestyle, it will be:

Sedentary Female = Female BMR x 1.2.

Daily Calorie Requirements for lightly active Male: Male BMR x 1.375

Lightly Female: Female BMR x 1.375

For moderately active Male: Male BMR x 1.55

Moderately active Female: Female BMR x 1.55

For very active male: Male BMR x 1.725

Very Active Female: Female BMR x 1.725

For Extra active male: Male BMR x 1.9

Extra active Female: Female BMR x 1.9

Classes of of Food, Sources and Functions

There are two major divisions of food namely, macronutrients and micronutrients, which comprise of four macronutrients, and two micronutrients. The macronutrients are listed as, carbohydrates, protein, fats and oil (lipids), and fibre (roughages) and the micronutrients are vitamins, and minerals plus trace elements. These classes of food are the suggestions of previous authors; however, to this author, there is one more class of food that is missing, and that is water. Water was never mentioned as a class of food in nutrition books but, since this author's 14 years of investigation on nutrition has suggested that water is an essential class of food, she is confident to mention and include water as the seventh class. The seven classes of food are five macronutrients namely, water, protein, carbohydrates, fats & oil, and fibre (roughages), and two micronutrients namely vitamins, and minerals plus trace elements. In this chapter, we will discuss about the macronutrients, their functions, food sources, and conditions that affect food metabolism.

Below are various types of food and its functions to the body:

Water (H20): (H+H+0).

Just like some physicians in Europe and North America do not consider water in providing prescription and medical advice, Nutrition authors are yet to mention or include water as vital macronutrient. Since the discovery of the criticality of water through desk research and water study intervention by this author, she was encouraged to include water in this book as a macronutrient MISSING in the macronutrient list until now. This author has used water or hydration to restore chronic health conditions to patients. She therefore, maintains that dehydration is directly connected with several health conditions. Thus, she dared to mention that water is a major component of macronutrient that has escaped great scholars and philosophers in health. A diet cannot be balanced without optimum consumption of water. Just like fat-soluble vitamins cannot be accessible to the body without fats and oil, water-soluble nutrients cannot be available to the body without sufficient amount of water in the body. Acute shortage of water or dehydration negatively affects the body metabolic processes and cause system breakdown, body malfunction and diseases. Adequate hydration promotes good metabolic processes, disposes the body to function properly and prevents diseases associated with dehydration such as Parkinson, constipation, poor bowel movement, nervous and muscle aches and breakdown as well as central nervous system, brain function, and more. To elaborate more on water, author created a separate chapter at the end of this book to educate the world more about water and the healing power of hydration and disease risks associated with shortage of water or dehydration.

Carbohydrates

Carbohydrates supply energy to the body, which is needed for daily activities. It comes in a complex form such as starch as well as in simple form example, sugar, glucose, honey, and fructose. Complex carbohydrates are generally healthier for the body than the simple ones. However, all simple sugars that are obtained from natural sources that are not processed are equally healthy food. For example, honey and fructose (fruit sugar). Complex carbohydrates could be referred to as starchy food and it mostly comes in natural forms. Examples of natural starchy foods are cassava, yam, potatoes, cereals, plantain, wheat, millet and cocoyam (17, 18, 20). The Recommended dietary allowance for carbohydrates is between 50% and 55%, and from two years and older 20g to 25g of dietary fibre is recommended daily for an individual (3, 5, 7, 16, 19, 20).

Dietary fibre (Roughages)

Dietary fibre are obtained from fruits, vegetables, whole grains, legumes, and nuts. They are the portion of the fibrous foods that cannot be digested by the body, and yet they play vital functions to the body. The gut or intestine bacterial need them to perform beneficial functions to the body. They aid weight loss and lower human risk of metabolic syndrome diseases. They are highly beneficial to health. Essential for digestion, cardiovascular system health, and metabolic processes. The food sources of roughages are often good sources of vitamins and minerals, which are essential for boosting and maintenance of body immunity to protect the body against diseases. Between 20g to 25g of fibre is daily recommendation for a person aged two years and above (3, 5, 7, 16, 19, 20, 73).

Protein

Protein is a type of food that is essential for growth, repair and replacing of dead cells and worn out tissues. All animal products are major sources of protein. Others are from the plant, and they occur mostly in legumes – all types of beans. However, animal protein is superior to plant's (3, 7, 16, 19, 20). It means that animal protein supplies comparatively superior (better) quality protein to the human body than plant protein. However, when beans are cooked together with corn, both offers each order the synergy that generates a product that matches closely with animal protein (16, 17, 18). Additionally, the consumption of whole wheat bread with peanut or peanut butter supplies the body the complete protein that it could obtain from animal protein (3, 7, 16,a; 19, 20); however, caution is highly required for peanut and peanut butter consumption because of its harmful polyunsaturated fatty acids, and lectin composition. About 10 to 35% of an individual's daily calories are recommended to be from protein. Please, note that peanut, and several sources of vegetable oil may not be the best for health.

Fat & Oil

Apart from being an excellent source of energy, it provides insulation and heat to the body. Without fat or oil, the body cannot utilize all the fat-soluble vitamins. Although, obesity and many health hazards are blamed on fats and cholesterol (if you would read my other book titled, *Nutrition for Chronic Diseases Prevention and Control* you will learn more about Cholesterol); fat and oil is essential for daily body metabolism and body upkeep. It is needed in every part and system of the human body. On this very note, those concerned about weight loss and high blood cholesterol must be careful not to eliminate oil entirely from their diet, they should rather use healthy fat and oil moderately, guided by professional advice.

Individuals with peculiar body situations and health conditions should seek professional help to make healthy choices of **types** of oil that are suitable. Fats and oil can be obtained from plants and animals namely, meat, poultry, fish, olive oil, linseed oil, cod liver oil, palm oil, groundnut oil, sunflower oil, cottonseed oil, coconut oil, sesame seed oil and other vegetable oil sources (5). It is worthy of note that not all of these oil sources are suitable for human consumption. Some have lectin, and some were hydrogenated, and refined. Lectin, hydrogenated, and refined oils and fats must be avoided to remain healthy. Fats and oils from Olive oil, mackerel, avocado pear, and egg yolks. Flaxseed, Salmon, walnut, and almond oils are also rich sources of Omega-3, which is healthy for the body. Without fat and oil, the vitamins A, D, E, and K (ADEK) cannot be absorbed or utilized by the body so, lipid is essential for ADEK absorption (3, 5, 7, 16, 17, 18, 20). Omega 3 and omega 6 are required in the body at a ratio of 4:1 that means, taking 4 grams of omega 3, and 1 gram of omega 6 is good to supply the body healthy fats/oil that it needs.

Conditions that Affects Food Metabolism

Derived from food consumption are substances known as: macronutrients, and micronutrients. Examples of macronutrients are: Carbohydrates, protein, fats and oil, and roughages (fibre). Examples of the micronutrients are vitamins, and minerals plus trace elements (5, 9). Food flavours, colours, and toxic substances namely, caffeine, steroids, cyanides, and salicylates affects the metabolism of the food.

The vitamin C level of the human body determines the level of iron derived from plants by a person, and the level of carbohydrates absorbed by the body is enhanced by the quantity of roughages ingested with the food (6).

For the human body to function efficiently, it requires a minimum amount of these seven categories of food in its daily meals. However, the choice of **specific** food that suit the complexities of different individuals' nature such as blood group, body mechanism and state of health, remains the bone of contention and issue of concern to people. Especially, as it concerns chronic diseases prevention and control. Examples of chronic diseases, which are also called metabolic syndrome diseases are, heart diseases, cancer, diabetes, obesity, overweight, hypothyroidism, and hyperthyroidism, rheumatism, and other health situations that are peculiar to individual (5, 9).

Body metabolism could be altered by disorders of the digestive system and gastrointestinal system (GIS), and defects of thyroid gland and hormone (11, 12, 13, 14). In some cases, it results into the inability of the body to digest lactose from milk. Others are peptic ulcer: causing the erosion of the duodenum, or stomach and celiac (sprue) disease, caused by excessive eating of wheat gluten. Too much of gluten destroys the lining of the small intestine called villi, and this result into the malabsorption of digested nutrients (9,11, 12, 13,14).

Other disorders of the digestive system are: diverticulosis, which is a protrusion of the belly caused by the development of small sacs in the large intestine. Colon polyps are another form of disorder caused by non-cancerous growth in the colon and the body. Polyps can grow in many parts of the body, and an extreme case could result in cancer (15,13). Polyps could be removed from the colon by a process called colonoscopy. It could occur as a consequence of an accessory organ disorders namely, hepatitis caused by viruses and toxins causing inflammation of the liver; malnutrition caused by under-eating or overeating causing nutrient excess of nutrients in the body and obesity. The United Nation's (UN) estimated records showed that 13% of the global population is undernourished, and 34% obese.

Question 1
How many major classes of food do we have? Name them.

Answer 1
There are two broad classes of food. They are macronutrients and micronutrients.

Question 2
How many classes are the macronutrients? Name them.

Answer 2
There are four traditional classes plus water making them five, namely, Carbohydrates, protein, lipids, fibre, and water.

Question 3
Why was water included by this author?

Answer 3
Researchers including this author have suggested in their various studies that dehydration is directly connected with several health conditions and this author have used

water or hydration to restore chronic health conditions to patients, including this author. With the lesson about macronutrients and conditions that affects metabolism, next, is a lesson about micronutrients overview.

Having learned about macronutrients, next, is a lesson about the micronutrients.

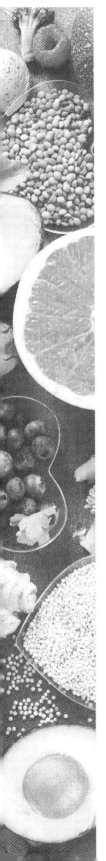

Chapter 2

Micronutrients Overview

Micronutrients constitute the vitamins, minerals plus trace elements. Vitamins are organic component that are essential for life and minerals are the inorganic component that are also necessary for health and well being. They are needed in the body in small quantity, compared to the macronutrients (6, 21, 22). Micronutrients are necessary for the production of enzymes, hormones, and other essential substances for all body metabolic processes, functions and upkeep (23). Micronutrients are essential in building strong bones, bodies and healthy brain. Micronutrients generally perform multiple functions in the body, often they are involved in more than one biochemical activities in the body (21). The absence of micronutrients can be very severe to the body and pose enormous threat to health. Lack of vitamin A, iodine, and iron pose significant threats to the body especially, in children and pregnant women (24). Lack of micronutrients result in birth defects such as, low birth weight, stillbirth and death. Others are cognitive delays, stunted growth, low immunity and susceptibility to diseases in children (25). Iodine deficiency causes preventable brain damage. Also, vitamin A deficiency weakens the immune system, affects the sight, makes children susceptible to measles and diarrhea (23). While minerals and vitamins are needed in small quantities in the body, trace elements are needed in minute quantities and yet their absence or deficiencies result in health problems. Vitamins and minerals essential for preventing and managing chronic diseases are highlighted below.

Vitamins

Vitamins are organic compounds found in food and are generally needed in small or trace amount in the body but, they perform different essential metabolic and biochemical functions in human body daily. Some of the organic compounds are not fully vitamins but, they are easily converted to vitamins by specific enzymes of the body. Those compounds are called provitamins or precursors. There are about 13 vitamins in the body, some are fat-soluble and some are water-soluble (3, 19). The body can manufacture some vitamins. Hence, they are called non-essential vitamins, and the body cannot produce some. The vitamins that the body cannot produce are called essential vitamins; meaning that a person needs to eat the food that contains it before the body can have and use it (19). While water remains the same in structure at all times, and carbohydrates, proteins, and fats have resemblance with one another, vitamins do not resemble each other. Vitamins are classified based upon their specific function to the body and based on characteristics or chemical composition (3, 19).

Except for choline, which is required in large amount in the body, vitamins are generally required in trace amount from micrograms (ug) to milligrams (mg) in the body daily, and yet, the body cannot function well or may break down without them. Like I stated earlier, some vitamins can be synthesized in the body, and some cannot. For example, vitamin D can be synthesized by ultraviolet light with precursor in human skin. This precursor is called niacin and it is made from a type of amino acid (protein) called tryptophan (3).

Vitamins therefore may be defined as complex organic compounds that occur naturally in food, plants, animals and nature, which are needed in human body in small amount and are essential for body metabolism, and excess, or lack of it can cause diseases to human body. Some vitamins are co-factors, meaning that they work together with other vitamins, or food, or mineral and enzymes to perform a specific function (1, 2, 3, 4, 19).

Lack of any vitamin, which the body cannot manufacture by itself can lead to a health problems and system malfunction. Examples of vitamins are vitamins A, B-group nine (9) of them (B1, B2, B3, B5, B6, B7, B8, B9, B12), C, D, E and K (1, 2, 3, 4, 19). Both B7 and B8 are called biotin.

Excessive intake of vitamins result in hypervitaminosis also called hypertoxicity of vitamins; a situation whereby vitamin is consumed excessively for a long period of time or in chronic situation. It could be consumed excessively for a short period of time to the point that it becomes harmful to the body. If the body lacks a particular vitamin for a long time it is called vitamin deficiency or hypovitaminosis and it results in illnesses (6, 21, 22). Excess or deficiencies can result in illnesses.

Vitamins Classification

Vitamins are placed into two major groups namely, fat-soluble vitamins and water-soluble vitamins. Fat soluble –means that vitamins under this group can only be dissolved and absolved in an oil solution. For example, Vitamin A, D, E and K. And water-soluble- meaning able to be dissolved and absorbed by the body in water solution. Examples, vitamin C and the nine B-group vitamins. Vitamins A, D, E and K are fat-soluble so, it is absorbed in the body in similar way dietary fats are absorbed in the body in the presence of bile and micelles or hydrophilic end of the fatty acids. They are excreted from human body from the bile through the feaces (3, 7, 19). Fat-soluble vitamins consist of carbon, hydrogen and oxygen.

Excess of fat-soluble vitamins like vitamins A and D have potentials to cause serious health problems. Water-soluble vitamins namely, Vitamins C and B-group vitamins are needed daily for body metabolism, and cannot be stored in the body, except vitamin B12, which can be stored in the body (3, 19). Water-soluble vitamin consist of carbon, hydrogen, oxygen, sulphur, cobalt and nitrogen. Excess of them is non-toxic and are excreted through the urine. It is important to note that there are compounds grouped as vitamins but the grouping is controversial example is **choline**, which is needed and synthesized in the body and are required in large amount and yet, it performs critical functions in the body to keep the body healthy.

Here is a list of fat-soluble and water-soluble vitamins:

Fat-soluble: There are four major fat-soluble vitamins namely, vitamins A and its vitamers, D and its vitamers,

E and its vitamers, and K and its vitamers. Vitamin A has two vitamers namely, Vitamins A1-retinol, and A2-dehydroretinol. Vitamin D has two vitamers namely, Vitamins D2-ergocalciferol, and D3-cholecalciferol. Vitamin E (tocopherol) has two major forms, the tocopherols and the tocotrienols and each has four vitamers namely, alpha-tocopherol, beta-tocopherol, gamma-tocopherol, and y-tocopherol, and alpha-tocotrienol, beta-tocotrienol, gamma-tocotrienol, and y-tocotrienol. Vitamin K has three vitamers namely, vitamins K1-phylloquinone, K2-melaquinone, and K3-menadione (3, 19).

Water-soluble: Vitamins B1-thiamin, B2-riboflavin, vitamin B3, or pp- niacin, vitamin B5- pantothenic acid, vitamins B6- pyridoxine, pyridoxal, pyridoxamine, vitamin B12-cobalamin, vitamin H-Biotin (B7 and B8), vitamin M (B9 and folacin), vitamin C-ascorbic acid, and choline-gossypine (3, 19).

Naming or Nomenclature of Vitamins

Vitamins were named based on the functions that they perform. Sometimes a vitamin that perform similar function may manifest different structures therefore, sometimes vitamins names were denoted with numbers for specific identification. example vitamins D2 and D3 (3,19). To do further clarity on the naming to make it easy for identification, vitamins were given names other than their chemical structures namely, riboflavin, thiamine, and niacin. Some naming were based upon source and function. Biotin, which is vitamin H was obtained from a German name for skin "haut". Vitamin K was obtained from a Danish name "koagulation", which means coagulation, and pantothenic acid was derived from a Greek word "pantos", which denotes "found everywhere" (3, 19). So vitamin B5, which is pantothenic acid occurs widely in plant and animal sources. Next, is the sources of vitamin.

Sources of Vitamins

Vitamins are generally obtained from plant, ultraviolet light from the sun, and animals can make some when they eat plant that contain the vitamins using animal digestive enzymes. B-group vitamins and K are manufactured in the large intestine from unabsorbed and undigested food (3,19). For example niacin is synthesized from a trip of protein- amino-acid called tryptophan found largely in turkey. While water-soluble vitamins are located or distributed to all parts of the body, fat-soluble vitamins do not occur in all parts of the body. They are located in specific parts of the body (3).

Questions 1
How many broad classes of vitamins do we have? What are their names?

Answer 1:
There are two major classes of vitamins. They are water-soluble vitamins and fat-soluble vitamins.

Question 2
How many major classifications of fat-soluble vitamins do we have?, Name them.

Answer 2
There are four major classes of fat-soluble vitamins namely, Vitamins A, D, E, and K.

Question 3
How many vitamers does each have?

Answer 3
There are two vitamers of Vitamin A, two vitamers of vitamin D, three vitamers of vitamins K. Vitamin E comes in two forms, tocopherols and tocotrienols and each has four vitamers each.

Question 4

How many major classifications of water-soluble vitamins do we have?, Name them.

Answer 4

There are two major classes of water-soluble vitamins namely, B-group vitamins and Vitamins C.

Question 5

How many B-group vitamins have we? Name them.

Answer 5

There are nine (9) B-group vitamins namely, vitamins B1, B2, B3, B5, B6, biotin (B7 and B8), B9 (folate), and B12 (cobalamin).

With the lesson about micronutrient overview in mind next, are specific lessons about fat-soluble vitamins starting with vitamin A.

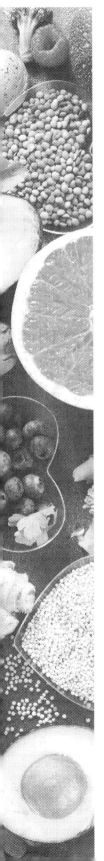

Chapter 3

Fat-Soluble vitamin: Vitamin A

Vitamin A was first identified as "accessory growth factor" it occurs in two major forms called vitamers namely Vitamins A1-retinol, and A2- dehydroretinol, and another form is carotene (alpha-, beta-, gamma-carotene, and cryptoxanthine (corn carotene)), which is known as precursor of vitamin A. Meaning that it is easily converted to vitamin A when consumed by animals to serve the same purpose as vitamin A (1, 2, 3, 4, 19). Beta carotene is more potent than the rest of other carotene, potency is close to that of vitamin A itself. Thus, one molecule of beta carotene equals one molecule of vitamin A. Sometimes carotene is not properly digested owing to certain factors.

Plants grown in winter period have low digestibility by animals but, the ones grown in warm climate or weather condition are more easily digested in the presence of its digestive enzymes examples beta carotene-15,15'-dioxyginase, which converts carotene first to retinaldehyde, and retinaldehyde reductase, which eventually reduces retinaldehyde to retinol (vitamin A) (25, 26). Therefore, the conversion of beta carotene to retinol involves redox (oxidation and reduction processes). Beta carotene is converted to vitamin A in the mucosa of the intestine, precisely, at the proximal jejunum. The lipid micelles acting as a carrier takes up vitamin A to mucosa cell from where it is diffused into the membrane of microvilli. Ninety percent (90%) of vitamin A is stored in the liver, the rest are stored in the blood, kidney, lungs and adrenal gland (1, 2, 3, 4, 19).

Functions of vitamin A

Growth: It is called a "growth factor" by early researchers cited in this book's vitamin literature because, when animals were not fed with food that has vitamin A, they did not grow well, and eventually, they died. But when animal experiencing poor growth were fed with vitamin A, the regained growth and survived. Therefore, vitamin A is an essential nutrient for young and growing animals and child bearing mothers (1, 2, 3, 4, 19).

Fertility and Reproduction: Vitamin A is essential for reproduction and reproductive health. It boost spermatozoa production and male reproductive function. Also, vitamin A promotes female reproductive function, ranging from estrogen, conception, retaining, and healthy growth of fetus in the female womb (1, 2, 3, 4, 19).

Vision: vitamin A is good for vision and general body well being. It promotes eye health, clear sight and it is good for the treatment of night blindness and conjuctivitis.

Bone: Vitamin A is essential for the formation and development of healthy bones including the cartilage.

Immune Booster: Vitamin A is a strong immune booster being an antioxidant. Vitamin A and all antioxidants have the potency for boosting the body immune system and protecting the body against infectious and chronic diseases invasion. Vitamin A protects the body from fungi, bacteria and viral diseases. It is potent against parasitic organisms examples, ringworm-*Trichophytonverrucosum*, hookworm, round worm and microbial organisms namely, staphylococcus aureus, and salmonella gallinarum. Vitamin A offers the body protection against cancer, psoriasis, and acne (1, 2, 3, 4).

Deficiency

Stunted Growth: Deficiency of vitamin A cause stunted growth-poor growth, and could cause death of the young including fetus in the womb.

Poor Fertility and Reproduction: It results into fertility problems, male and female reproductive problems, by causing poor or unhealthy genital epithelial cells. It cause a degeneration of male epithelial and seminiferous tubules and cessation of sperm production, leading to poor or low sperm count and spermatozoa production, and low sexual activities. It lowers testosterone. It can cause abortion or death of fetus (baby in the womb) (1, 2, 3, 4, 7,19). It can affect egg formation in female, including the quantity and size of egg.

Vision problems: Deficiency of vitamin A causes poor sight, night blindness, and eye diseases. Loss of lens, constriction of optic nerve and other kind of eye diseases or defects.

Bone Problems: Vitamin A is good for bone development and bone health, therefore, deficiency of vitamin A results in all bone associated diseases namely, osteoporosis, disorganized growth of the bone, and irritation of the joint, nervous problem and pressure in the cerebellum fluid (1, 2, 3, 4, 19).

Weak Immunity: Vitamin A is a powerful immune booster as an antioxidant so, deficiency of vitamin A results in poor or weak immune system. Deficiency of vitamin A and all antioxidants result to poor immune system and exposing the body against infectious and chronic diseases invasion. Vitamin A protects the body from fungi, bacteria and viral diseases, so its deficiency exposes the body to these microbial attack. It is potent against ringworm-*Trichophytonverrucosum*, hookworm, round worm, staphylococcus aureus, and salmonella gallinarum, again its deficiency can expose the body to their susceptivity (1, 2, 3, 4, 7, 19). It can cause a restriction of brain functions. It can cause edema, unhealthy and untidy hair. Deficiency of vitamin A can cause cyst (abnormal growth) in the pituitary gland, diarrhea and loss of appetite (1, 2, 3, 4, 19).

Liver: deficiency of vitamin A can cause liver malfunction.

Nervous System Problems: It can cause a range of nervous problem including high pressure on cerebrospinal fluid, and nerve twisting.

Respiratory System problem: Vitamin A deficiency can cause respiratory diseases namely, lung abscesses, nasal discharge, and pneumonia.

Urinary System problems: It can cause urinary diseases including Cystitis, Nephrosis, pus in the ureters, pyelitis, urolithiasis, and bladder wall thickening (1, 2, 3, 4, 19).

Toxicity

Excessive intake of vitamin A or overdose results in hypervitaminosis of vitamin A. It can manifest in loss of skeletal bone, loss of appetite, internal hemorrhage, loss of weight and thickening of the skin. Others are low keratinization, rapid blood clotting, slow growth, fragile liver, low red blood cell count, conjunctivitis, congenital abnormalities, degenerative atrophy, low liver and kidney functions, and pelvic fins. It can cause abnormal bone modelling, causing fractures, short bone formation, and retarded growth, and weakening of cell membranes (1, 2, 3, 4, 19).

An elevated level of vitamin A, 200 ug per decilitre above normal in children cause intracranial problem-high pressure in the cerebrospinal fluid (CSF) inside the skull, and dermatological problems namely, pyritic skin rash, hydrocephalous-Accumulation of CSF in the brain, causing pain in the legs and arms of children (1, 2, 3, 4, 19).

Requirements

Lactating Mothers: 1,200 ug/RE
Children: 400-700 ug RE
Adult: 800-1000 ug/RE
ug: Microgram; RE: Retinol equivalent

Sources of Vitamin A

Palm fruit or fresh unadulterated palm Oil, plantain, fish liver, fish oil, liver, Halibut liver oil, cod liver oil, egg yolk, carrot, fresh tomatoes, red pepper, milk, green plants, and legumes. Others are butter. The greener the plant the more its carotene content (7, 8).

Stability

Vitamin A is unstable when exposed to oxidation, light (photoxidation) and at high temperature in the presence of oxygen. However, if heated at high temperature without oxygen, the denaturing and depleting of vitamin A is minimized (not much), Curing (salting, drying and smoking) of carotene or vitamin A source, these processes can lead to a loss of up to 80%. Butter exposed to 50 degrees Centigrade loses its vitamin A completely, conversely, when it is exposed to 120 degrees Centigrade in absence of oxygen, it is not lost (7; 8).

Vitamins A, C, D and E are powerful sources of antioxidant. Meaning that they are vitamins that protects the body cells from decay or oxidation. Oxidative activities inside the human body triggers lots of diseases in the body including, coronary heart diseases, formation of cancer cells, weakening of liver and pancreatic functions including, ineffective insulin secretion and or low insulin secretion (19, 27).

On set of body cell oxidation results in diseases associated with metabolic syndrome such as, high blood sugar, diabetes, high blood cholesterol, overweight, obesity, cancer, arthritis, coronary and pulmonary heart diseases, and thyroid stimulating hormone problem (27). Advanced case of cell oxidation can result in gut leakage. Also, animals with injured blood vessels that had their peroxide level raised by 2.5 fold than normal after two weeks of sustaining the injury; after treating them with vitamins C and E both separately and combined, the animals showed significant reduction in the formation of peroxides in the injured coronary arteries, was beneficial to healing and recovery because it lowered the oxidative stress level of the blood vessels (27).

Women who have passed menopause were treated with hormone replacement therapy (HRT). Some of them have diabetes type II and some do not. Half of the ones with diabetes type II and those without diabetes received both HRT and vitamins C and E (VCE) only throughout the treatment period and half received HRT only (28). The result showed that the diabetic ones manifested a significant rise of red blood cell count called glycated haemoglobin (HbA1c). Change also occurred in the white blood cell count, vitamin A, and high density lipoprotein (cholesterol) but, it was not significant (not much) (28).

Those treated with HRT and VCE also manifested reduction in blood sugar level, and platelet. And rise in blood vitamin E, carotenoid level, catalase, glutathione peroxidase ((7, 8, 28). Presence of glutathione peroxidase cause a reduction in red blood cell and plasma glutathione level of the blood. The summary is that the treatment of postmenopausal women both diabetic and non diabetic resulted in the reduction of blood sugar and cholesterol levels as well as rise in blood antioxidants level and metabolic enzymes (28).

Question 1
What are the functions of vitamin A to the body?

Answer 1
Optimum consumption of vitamin A is beneficial to the following:

Growth: It is called a "growth factor", when animals were not fed with food that has vitamin A, they did not grow well, and eventually, they died. But when animal experiencing poor growth were fed with vitamin A, the regained growth and survived. Therefore, vitamin A is an essential nutrient for young and growing animals and child bearing mothers.

Fertility and Reproduction: Vitamin A is essential for reproduction and reproductive health. It boost spermatozoa production and male reproductive function. Also, vitamin A promotes female reproductive function, ranging from estrogen, conception, retaining, and healthy growth of fetus in the female womb.

Vision: vitamin A is good for vision and general body health. It promotes eye health, clear sight and good for the treatment of night blindness and conjuctivitis.

Bone: Vitamin A is essential for the formation, development and health bone including the cartilage.

Immune Booster: Vitamin A is a powerful immune booster being an antioxidant. Vitamin A and all antioxidants have the potency for boosting the body immune system and protecting the body against infectious and chronic diseases invasion. Vitamin A protects the body from fungi, bacteria and viral diseases. It is potent against ringworm-*Trichophytonverrucosum*, hookworm, round worm, staphylococcus aureus, and salmonella gallinarum.

Question 2
What are the consequences of deficiency of vitamin A?

Answer 2
When the body is deficient in vitamin A, the following will be the consequence:

Stunted Growth: Deficiency of vitamin A cause stunted growth-poor growth, and could cause death of the young including fetus in the womb.

Poor Fertility and Reproduction: It results into fertility problems, male and female reproductive problems, by causing poor or unhealthy genital epithelial cells. It cause a degeneration of male epithelial and seminiferous tubules and cessation of sperm production, leading to poor or low sperm count and spermatozoa production, and low sexual activities. It lowers testosterone. It can cause abortion or death of fetus (baby in the womb). It can affect egg formation in female, including the quantity and size of egg.

Vision problems: Deficiency of vitamin A causes poor sight, night blindness, and eye diseases. Loss of lens, constriction of optic nerve and other kind of eye diseases or defects.

Bone Problems: Vitamin A is good for bone development and bone health, therefore, deficiency of vitamin A results in all bone associated diseases namely, osteoporosis, disorganized growth of the bone, and irritation of the joint, nervous problem and pressure in the cerebellum fluid (1, 2, 3, 4, 19).

Weak Immunity: Vitamin A is a powerful immune booster as an antioxidant so, deficiency of vitamin A results in poor or weak immune system. Deficiency of vitamin A and all antioxidants result to poor immune system and exposing the body against infectious and chronic diseases invasion. Vitamin A protects the body from fungi, bacteria and viral diseases, so its deficiency exposes the body to these microbial attack. It is potent against ringworm-*Trichophytonverrucosum*, hookworm, round worm, staphylococcus aureus, and salmonella gallinarum, again its deficiency can expose the body to their susceptivity. Vitamin A offers the body protection against cancer, psoriasis, and acne.

Restriction of brain functions: It can cause edema, unhealthy and untidy hair. It can cause cyst (abnormal growth) in the pituitary gland, diarrhea and loss of appetite.

Liver: deficiency of vitamin A can cause liver malfunction.

Nervous System Problems: It can cause a range of nervous problem including high pressure on cerebrospinal fluid, and nerve twisting.

Respiratory System problem: Vitamin A deficiency can cause respiratory diseases namely, lung abscesses, nasal discharge, and pneumonia.

Urinary System problems: It can cause urinary diseases including Cystitis, Nephrosis, pus in the ureters, pyelitis, urolithiasis, and bladder wall thickening.

Keeping in thoughts the lesson about vitamin A next, is about Vitamin D.

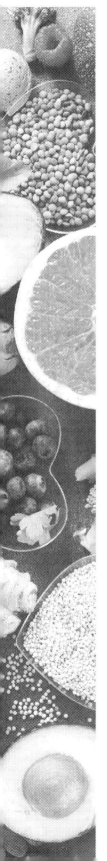

Chapter 4

Fat-Soluble vitamin: Vitamin D (Sunshine vitamin)

Vitamin D is called sunshine vitamin because it is manufactured or synthesized by plants and animals when they are exposed to sufficient sunlight. Vitamin D occurs in two main forms Vitamins D2-ergocalciferol that are obtained predominantly from plant, and D3-cholecalciferol, the one obtained from animals (7, 8). Vitamin D is not needed in diet or supplement if one is exposed to sufficient sunlight. Also, food namely butter and milk when irradiated gained vitamin D from irradiation with ultraviolet light and children fed with irradiated milk and butter did not suffer rickets again (3, 7, 8, 29, 30, 31).

When the bone cannot mineralize, the consequence is rickets in children and osteomalacia in adult. This might be a message of hope for people who are concerned about food irradiation that irradiated food could provide a much needed vitamin D, although, it could lead to loss of some other nutrients namely, vitamins A, C and heat sensitive nutrients. Vitamin D can also function as a hormone Vitamins D2-ergocalciferol, and D3-cholecalciferol (7, 8, 30).

Vitamin D is located anywhere there is sunshine, and also in the blood, kidney, liver, and lungs, with blood containing the highest amount of vitamin D followed by the liver. Vitamin D performs many functions in the body but, the main functions are, to absorb, metabolize, retain, and deposit calcium and phosphorus to the bones. Vitamin D also, performs a hormone function aside being a mineral. It resembles steroid hormone in its function. Vitamin D is manufactured inside the body by liver and kidneys. Kidney is the main site where vitamin D is synthesized in the body (7, 8, 33, 34, 35).

Vitamin D is a form of hormone produced in human and animal skin by a process called photolysis from vitamin D called 7-dehydrocholesterol to perform hormonal function and regulation. When hydrogen is removed from vitamin D (dehydrogenation process) steroid is formed out of it. Other than being produced in the skin by sunshine, when cod liver oil or fish oil was moderately irradiated (7, 8, 31), it boosted the body immune system, and it was good for healthy skin (33, 34, 35). It also protect the body cell from malignant actions of cancer and it prevents cancer development, and it is believed that more health benefits are yet to unfold from vitamin D benefits to human and animal bodies (33, 34, 35).

Vitamin D manufactured in the liver is called metabolites 25-hydroxyvitamin D3 (25-OHD3), it can also be manufactured by chemical process and it could be metabolized in the body to serve a purpose of vitamin D. Vitamin D has precursors namely, ergosterol, and 7-dehydrocholesterol. Vitamin D3-cholecalciferol is manufactured from animal products, and 7-dehydrocholesterol is produced inside the body from cholesterol or squalene, and it is predominantly located under the skin, walls of the intestine and other tissues (7, 8, 29, 30, 31).

Vitamin D is destroyed when over irradiated with ultraviolet light, or peroxidation of polyunsaturated fatty acid has gone rancid. Antirachitic function (prevention of rickets) of vitamin D comes on only after ultraviolet irradiation (7, 8). Irradiation of rats suffering from rachitic or irradiated food given to them showed presence of vitamin D, which did not show prior to irradiation or feeding with irradiated food. About 0.025 microgram (ug) of vitamin D3 equals one United States Pharmacopeial Convention (USP) of vitamin D function. Simply **rubbing cod liver oil on the skin of a child with rickets and exposing to ultraviolet light** is enough to heal or treat the rickets (7, 8).

Vitamin D therefore could be consumed orally or synthesized in the epidermis of the skin by photochemical process called photolysis, and transported to the intestine and bone through the blood. Up to 90%

of precursor of vitamin D is located under the epidermal layer of the skin. Before vitamin D is utilized by the body, it undergoes a series of transformation (3, 7, 33). Vitamin D circulating in the blood do so slowly and in low concentration; hence, why vitamin D accumulates in the liver rapidly. In the liver, vitamin D undergoes chemical changes, which involves chromosomal hydrolysis. The product is a metabolite called 25-OH vitamin D (36; 37, 29, 30, 31).

Precursor of vitamin D. Although, the conversion of vitamin D3 to 25-OHD3 occurs largely in the chromosomes, its conversion enzyme is of low-capacity high-affinity metabolite- small or intermediate molecules formed after metabolism of vitamin D (3, 7, 38). Conversion also, happens in the mitochondria, and at mitochondria, the conversion enzyme is of high-capacity low-affinity. Mitochondria conversion occurs in time of vitamin D toxicity (3). A major hydroxylation of vitamin D occurs in the liver. Also minor hydroxylation of vitamin D occurs in the kidney and intestine.

Excretion of Vitamin D

Excretion: Bile salt aids in the excretion of vitamin D and its metabolites, through the feaces. Vitamin D that is absorbed in the blood can circulate for a maximum of 10 days, after which, it will begin to catabolize-break down in readiness for excretion.

Joint Functions of Vitamin D and Calcium and With Phosphorus

One of the general functions of vitamin D is to elevate calcium and phosphorus level in the blood to promote the mineralization-absorption of mineral by the bone and other parts of the body. It regulates the immune system of the body (30). Vitamin D is effective for treating leukaemia and psoriasis (33). **Significance reduction of blood calcium level below normal results in tetanus**. Vitamin D works jointly, and yet delicately with two enzymes namely, thyrocalcitonin, which is also called calcitonin and parathyroid hormone (PTH) to control the levels of calcium and phosphorus in the blood. Calcitonin performs three function to regulate high blood calcium namely, lowering its absorption in the gut, stopping bone demineralization, and prompting the kidney to reabsorb vitamin D (7, 8, 29, 30, 31).

Question
1. How does vitamin D regulate calcium and phosphorus levels in the Blood?

Answer:
Vitamin D works jointly with two enzymes called thyrocalcitonin and parathyroid hormone to regulate calcium and phosphorus concentrations in the blood.

2. What are the three functions that calcitonin performs to regulate high blood calcium in the blood?

Answer: The three functions performed by calcitonin or thyrocalcitonin to reduce high blood calcium are:

i.   It reduces the gut absorption of calcium.
ii. It stops demineralization of bone, and
iii. It signals the kidney to reabsorb vitamin D

On the other hand, vitamin D can raise serum phosphorus and calcium levels by simply stimulating the intestine, bone, and kidney to pump phosphorus and calcium into the blood to mineralize the bone and support calcium to perform its functions in the body (7, 8, 33).

Effect on Intestine: Vitamin D stimulates movement of calcium and phosphorus to the epithelium of the intestine. In times of hypocalcemia-low calcium absorption, parathyroid hormone stimulates the production of hydrolyzed vitamin D (1, 25-(OH)2D3 to prompt its absorption (7, 8, 26).

Effect on Bone: Vitamin D promotes the opposite functions to the bone namely, mineralization of bone, and demineralization of bone. Causing the bone to absorb calcium and phosphorus when they are needed, and also, causing the bone to stop mineral absorption when there is excess of them in circulation (7, 8).

Before vitamin D is utilized in the body, it is converted to vitamin D metabolites, and the vitamin D produced in the liver is a metabolite of vitamin D. There are up to 33 metabolites of vitamin D example

1,25-(OH)2D3. Also, 24,25-dihydroxyvitamin D3 is another functional vitamin D metabolite. It was suggested that when 24-position of vitamin D metabolite of 25-OH-D3 is replaced with flour groups it inhibits 24-hyroxylation and when this happens the formed compound is suggested to provide health benefit for up to two generations (26, 33, 29, 30, 31).

Deficient of Vitamin D

Vitamin D deficiency results in rickets in children, osteomalacia-demineralization (inhibiting mineral absorption), and osteoporosis in adult (7, 8, 32).

Required Range for the body

About 25-35 ng - nanogram, which is the same as 62-88 nmolar for a meal per a day is suggested as normal range, and for protection against degenerative diseases up tp 75-90 ng per meal is suggested to be desirable range (32).

Keeping in thoughts the lesson about vitamin D, next, is about vitamin E.

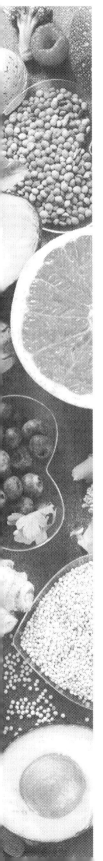

Chapter 5

Fat-Soluble Vitamin E: Anti-Fertility Factor

With the discovery of required factors namely, vitamins A, C, D, and thiamin and feeding animals with purified macronutrients namely, carbohydrates, protein, and required newly discovered vitamins, it was soon observed that though, the animals were doing well, and yet, both male and female animals recorded abnormally low fertility, so, they were not doing well reproductively. The male animals suffered degenerated testicle, and the female experienced impaired placenta hence, the females could not carry babies to full term (7, 8, 40).

Additionally, female suffered degeneration of smooth muscles of the uterus and both suffered degeneration of skeleton. The fertility diseases suffered by the animals were reversed when un-purified yeasts and fresh lettuce were added to the animals' feed. To distinguish fat-soluble vitamins A, and D from the new X factor that reversed infertility or fertility problem in the animals, when the animals were given vitamins A and D, the fertility problem existed; but, when the new discovered X factor was added to the animal feed, fertility was restored (7, 8, 41).

Cod liver oil that is high in vitamins A and D when given to the animal could not restore fertility, but, administering a single droplet of wheat germ oil every day prevented resorption in pregnant rat (death of fetus in mother's womb after organ formation). Then, the x factor that restored fertility was named vitamin E (7, 8, 19, 41). It was later discovered that that vitamin is also a powerful antioxidant.

Also, from unsaponifiable wheat germ lipid came a discovery of allophanic acid esters with three alcohol that perform the same biological function as vitamin E. It was later described as having phytyl side chain and a portion of hydroquinone, which described the chemical structure of vitamin E and named it tocopherol from a Greek words *tokos* meaning "childbirth", and pherein meaning "to bear" "ol" indicates that the x factor contains alcohol, and in fact, three molecules of alcohol, which forms the vitamers such as, alpha-, beta- and gamma- (g). Later, alpha-tocopherol were discovered from soy bean oil (7, 8, 19, 41), and and y-tocopherol was discovered. With more studies, a second vitamer of vitamin E was discovered called tocotrienols, and in the end vitamin E has two vitamers namely, the tocopherol, and tocotrienol, and they now have four vitamers each. Tocopherol vitamers are, alpha-tocopherol, beta-tocopherol, gamma-tocopherol, and y-tocopherol, and tocotrienol vitamers are, alpha-tocotrienol, beta-tocotrienol, gamma-tocotrienol, and y-tocotrienol.

Food Sources of Vitamin E and How to Determine Quantity and Daily Value (DV) in Each Source

Here is a list of food sources of vitamin E. In this list, the sources of vitamin E were mentioned, and a clue about how to determine the quantity of vitamin E that is in each source was also included.

Wheat germ oil: 1 teaspoon = 20mg =135% DV; 100 g = 149 mg = 996% DV.

Sunflower seeds: 1 ounce (28.35 g) =10 mg = 66% DV; 100g = 35 mg = 234% DV.

Almonds: 1 ounce (28.35 g) = 7.3 mg = 48% DV, 100 g = 26 mg = 171% DV.

Mamey sapote: Half fruit = 5.9 mg = 39% DV; 100 g = 2.1 mg = 14% DV.

Hazel nut: 1 ounce (28.35 g) = 4.3 mg = 28% DV; 100 g = 15 gm = 100% DV.

Ground nut or peanut: 1 ounce (28.35 g) = 2.4 mg = 16% DV; 100 g = 8.4 mg = 56% DV.

Egg 1 egg = 15% DV

Avocado pear: Half fruit: 2.1 mg = 14% DV; 100 g = 2.1 mg = 14% DV.

Atlantic Salmon: Half fillet = 2.0 mg = 14% DV; 100 g = 1.1 mg = 8% DV.

Rainbow trout (fish): 1 fillet = 2.0 mg = 13% DV; 100 g = 2.8 mg = 19% DV.

Raw red sweet bell pepper: 1 medium = 1.9 mg = 13% DV; 100 g = 1.6 mg = 11% DV.

Brazil nur: 1 ounce (28.35 g) = 1.6 mg = 11% DV; 100 g = 5.7 mg = 38% DV.

Mango: Half mango = 1.5 mg = 10% DV; 100 g - 0.9 mg = 6% DV.

Snail: 1 ounce (28.35 g) = 1.1 mg = 9% DV; 100 g = 5.0 mg = 33% DV.

Crayfish: 3 ounces (85.05) = 1.3 mg = 8% DV; 100 g = 1.5 mg = 10% DV.

Kiwi fruit: 1 medium size = 1.0 mg = 7% DV; 100 g = 1.5 mg = 10% DV.

Octopus: 3 ounces (85.05) = 1.0 mg = 7% DV; 100 g = 1.2 mg = 8% DV.

Black berries: half cup = 0.8 mg = 6% DV; 100 g = 1.2 mg = 8% DV.

Lobster: 3 ounces (85.05) = 0.9 mg = 6% DV; 100 g = 1.0 mg = 7% DV.

Dry Cod (Igbo name: okporoko): 1 ounce = 0.8 mg = 5% DV; 100 g = 2.8 mg = 19% DV.

Pistachios: 1 ounce (28.35 g) = 0.8 mg = 5% DV; 100 g = 2.9 mg = 19% DV.

Pumpkin seed/melon seed (igbo name egwusi): 1 ounce = 0.6 mg = 4% DV; 100 g = 2.2 mg = 15% DV.

Paw paw, 100 g = 4% DV.

Pecans: 0.4 mg = 3% DV; 100 g = 1.4 mg = 9% DV.

Cashew nuts: 1 ounce (28.35 g) = 0.3 mg = 2% DV; 100 g = 0.9 mg = 6% DV (7, 19, 41).

From the list above, you can see that the highest quantity of vitamin E was found in wheat germ oil, which contains 135% of DV per 20 milligram of wheat germ oil. The next high concentration source is Sunflower seeds with 66% DV obtainable from 28.35 g, which is equivalent to 1 ounce or 10 mg of vitamin E. Next, is Almonds, which is 1 ounce or 28.35 g, it contains 48% DV or 7.3 mg of vitamin E. The least amount of vitamin E and DV was found in cashew nut.

Please note that DV means daily value. DV: Daily value.

Questions
1. What was the X factor that reversed infertility or prevented fertility problem, which is neither vitamin A nor vitamin D?

Answer 1
It is called Vitamin E.

Question 2

When vitamins A and D could not restore fertility and a single droplet of wheat germ oil was administered, what diseases did it prevent?

Answer 2

It prevented resorption in pregnant rat and restored fertility.

With the lesson about vitamin E in mind, next, is about vitamin K.

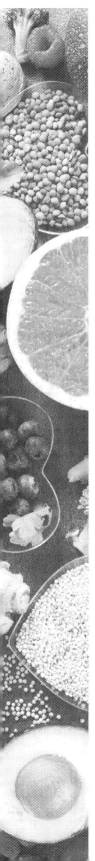

Chapter 6

Fat-Soluble vitamin:Vitamin K: Anti-hemorrhage Factor and Its Discovery

Vitamin K is a fat-soluble vitamin that contains prothrombin, which it uses to promote blood clot. Vitamin K is a vitamin that prevents anemia, hemorrhage and delayed blood clot. Vitamin K was discovered in 1929 when researchers fed chickens with animal feed that had its steroid extracted or removed. The feeding of chickens with animal feed without steroid resulted in chicken diseases that caused chicken to develop subdural, subcutaneous or intramuscular hemorrhages, anemia and delayed blood clotting (7, 42). Whereas the chickens that were given animal feed such as fish meal that contains steroid did not experience defect or delay in blood clotting, anemia or hemorrhage at all. Also chicken fed with cabbage achieved the same inhibition of blood clotting syndrome. It was also, observed that some component of plants and leaves and vegetables that is not vitamins A, C, D, and E was responsible for preventing blood clotting syndrome (7, 42).

It was called vitamin K. It was discovered that prothrombin was the blood clotting factor. The blood clotting syndrome experienced by chicken that were deficient in vitamin K that have partially purified blood prothrombin also showed depressed concentration of blood prothrombin (7, 42). When they were fed with vitamin K rich food, anemia, hemorrhage and delayed blood clot stopped, and normal blood clotting resumed and anemia and hemorrhage disappeared.

Just to make it clear that the story about how nutrients were discovered was meant to help all understand clearly that the lessons about the nutrients were not myths but facts that assist people to understand the connection between the nutrients and health and well being of both humans and lower animals as this author indicated from the beginning of the this book.

Functions

Optimum vitamin K in the body prevents delayed blood clotting, and promotes blood clotting. It also, prevents, anemia and hemorrhage in humans. In chicken, optimum vitamin K consumption prevented chicken from developing diseases such as subdural, subcutaneous or intramuscular hemorrhages, anemia and delayed blood clotting (7, 42).

Deficiency

Deficiency of vitamin K results in delayed blood clotting, anemia and hemorrhage in humans. In chicken, vitamin K deficiency caused chicken to develop subdural, subcutaneous or intramuscular hemorrhages, anemia and delayed blood clotting (7, 42).

Food Sources of Vitamin K

Putrified fish meals, animal feed with steroid, vegetables, leaves, cabbage are good sources. It could also be manufactured in the large intestine from undigested food (7, 42).

Vitamin K has vitamers namely, vitamin K1, K2, and K3. All can be synthesized

Question 1
1. What happened to chick fed with animal feed that has its steroid removed?

Answer 1

The chick suffered from subdural, intramuscular hemorrhages, anemia, and delayed blood clotting

Question 2

What happened to the chick fed with animal feed that its steroid was not removed, or chick fed with putrified fish meals, vegetables, leaves, or cabbage?

Answer 2

They neither suffered from subdural, subcutaneous hemorrhages, anemia, nor delayed blood clotting

Question 3

What was the anti-hemorrhage factor that prevented subdural, subcutaneous hemorrhage, anemia, and delayed blood clot called?

Answer 3

It is called vitamin K.

With the lesson about vitamin K in mind next, is about water-soluble vitamins beginning with B-group vitamin.

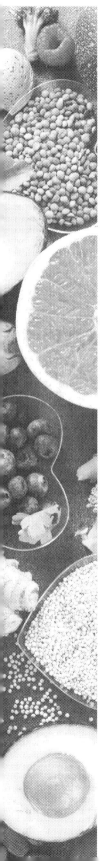

Chapter 7

Water-Soluble Vitamins: B-Group Vitamins

B-group vitamins are water-soluble vitamins that range from B1 - B12, which are needed in the body in small quantity, but are essential to health and well being.

Vitamin B1: Thiamine

It is a water-soluble vitamin, needed in the body in small amount and yet, it is essential to life. The importance of B1 in human diet was not discovered until 1884 by Chinese medicine that discovered high rate of death and illnesses among Japanese sailors; reason being polished rice and processed foods while on long sea journey. As soon as the sailors were placed on vegetables, whole grain, meat, and beans diet, their diseases vanished and death rate became low (7, 39, 44, 67). A little is stored in the liver so, more is required to be consumed for the body to have it. It occurs naturally on plant and animal sources alike (7, 39, 44).

Function

Vitamin B1 (thiamin) is essential for growth and cell activities.

Deficiency.

Result in high frequency of illnesses and high death rate. Heart and brain problems, and low energy supply to the body cell (7, 39, 44).

Source

Plant: Fresh vegetables, whole grains, beans, yam, coco yam, brown parboiled rice, lentils, green peas, and whole grain bread.

    Animal: Fish, and meat. Thiamine is located in the grain bran or outer covering after the shell or coat is removed (7, 39, 44, 67).

    Keeping in mind the lesson about B1 next, is about B2.

Riboflavin - Vitamin B2

Riboflavin is a water-soluble vitamin that occurs in plant-based and animal based food. Also, gut bacteria can produce small quantity of Riboflavin. **Coenzymes involved in energy production, cell growth, lipids breakdown (Digestion), digestion of medicines and steroids can not perform these functions without riboflavin** (7, 38, 42). It cannot be stored in the body, excess is removed from the body through the urine. It gives yellow colour to urine (7, 40, 44, 68).

Recommended Dietary Allowance (RDA)

RDA for B2 for female 19 and above is 1.1 mg per day, and male aged 19 years and above is 1.3 mg per day. Pregnant women 1.4 mg per day, and lactating mothers 1.6 mg per day (7, 40, 44).

Functions

Coenzymes involved in energy production, cell growth, lipids breakdown (Digestion), digestion of medicines and steroids can not perform these functions without riboflavin (7, 40, 44).

Deficiency

Health problems such as cancer, heart and brain disorders.

Sources

Plant: spinach, almonds.

Animal: Fish, milk and dairy products, lean - beef, chicken, and pork, cheese, eggs, organ meat - liver (7, 40, 44, 68).

With the lesson about B2 in thoughts next, is about B3.

Niacin: Vitamin B3

Niacin is a water-soluble vitamins that occurs naturally in some foods. In some cases it is added to some foods, and it is available as food supplement. Niacin comes in two forms namely, nicotinic acid and nicotinamide. Human body cannot store it thus, excess of it is excreted through urination (7, 8, 45). A brain-healthy amino acid called tryptophan can also be converted to nicotinamide. Niacin is a coenzyme, which is involved in over 400 enzyme functions. It exhibits anti-oxidation effect to the body cells. It is involved in DNA repairs, cholesterol and lipids production, and in conversion of nutrients into energy (7, 8, 45).

Functions

Niacin is a coenzyme, which is involved in over 400 enzyme functions. It exhibits anti-oxidation effect to the body cells. It is involved in DNA repairs, cholesterol and lipids production, and in conversion of nutrients into energy (7, 44, 45).

Recommended Dietary Allowance (RDA)

Counted as niacin equivalents (NE), and measured in mg. Sixty (60) mg of tryptophan is equal to one NE. For adults aged 19 years old and above female requires 14 mg NE per a day, and male requires 16 mg daily. Lactating mothers require 17 mg NE daily and pregnant women require 18 mg NE daily (7, 8, 45).

Deficiency

Niacin deficiency and all associated niacin functions will be hampered. As a coenzyme, it will hamper over 400 enzyme functions that niacin performs. It will increase cell oxidation because its anti-oxidation function will be inhibited. Its capacity to repair DNA will be inhibited, also. It will inhibit cholesterol and lipids production, and its capacity to convert nutrients

Sources

Plant sources: Brown parboiled rice, nuts, seeds, legumes, bananas, and whole grain bread.

    Animal sources: Fish, poultry, red meat, port, beef and beef liver (7, 8, 45).

Question 1
What are the functions of niacin to the body?

Answer 1
The following are the functions of vitamin B3:

Functions

Niacin is a coenzyme, and it is involved in over 400 enzyme functions. It exhibits anti-oxidation effect to the body cells. It is involved in DNA repairs, cholesterol and lipids production, and in conversion of nutrients into energy.

Question 2
What will happen to a body that is deficient in niacin?

Answer 2
Deficiency of niacin will result in the following:

Deficiency

Niacin deficiency and all associated niacin functions will be hampered. As a coenzyme, it will hamper over 400 enzyme functions that niacin performs. It will increase cell oxidation because its anti-oxidation function will be inhibited. Its capacity to repair DNA will be inhibited, also. It will inhibit cholesterol and lipids production, and its capacity to convert nutrients into energy (7, 8, 45).

Question 3
What is the recommended dietary allowance (RDA) for niacin?

Answer 3
The RDA for niacin is as follows:

Recommended Dietary Allowance (RDA)

Counted as niacin equivalents (NE), and measured in mg. Sixty (60) mg of tryptophan is equal to one NE. For adults aged 19 years old and above female requires 14 mg NE per a day, and male requires 16 mg daily. Lactating mothers require 17 mg NE daily and pregnant women require 18 mg NE daily (7, 8, 45).

Having learned about B3 next, is a lesson about B5.

Pantothenic acid - Vitamin B5

Like other B-group vitamins Pantothenic acid is a water-soluble vitamin that occurs naturally in plants and animal food. Just like vitamin B2, B5 can be produced in the human body by gut bacteria, although the quantity produced is small, not enough for body daily need so, more is required to be consumed. B5 is involved in the formation of coenzyme A (CoA). CoA is a chemical compound involved in other metabolic activities in the body and it is responsible for production and digestion of fatty acids (7, 8, 46).

Functions

B5 is involved in the formation of coenzyme A (CoA). CoA is a chemical compound involved in other metabolic activities in the body and it is responsible for production and digestion of fatty acids. It reduces the body cholesterol, low density lipoprotein (LDL)- bad cholesterol, and triglycerides, and it causes rise in good cholesterol called high density cholesterol (HDL). Some studies suggested that it lowers inflammation at early stage, and that it acts as antioxidant (7, 8, 46).

Recommended Dietary Allowance (RDA)

Adults aged 19 years old and above male and female requires only 5 mg per day. Pregnant women require 6 mg per day and lactating mother 7 mg per a day (7, 8, 46).

Deficiency

B5 deficiency is rare to see a person with vitamin B5 deficiency because it occurs everywhere. Malnutrition can cause it and a person that have problems digesting vitamin B5. It can cause headache, disturbed sleep, fatigue, muscle cramps, numbness or burning sensation in feet and hands, irritability, and restlessness (7, 8, 46).

Sources

Plant sources: Nuts, seeds, potatoes, mushrooms, brown parboiled rice, broccoli, yam, coco yam, oats, and avocado.

Animal: Chicken breast, milk and dairy products, yogurt, egg, beef, and organ meat (7, 8, 46).

Question 1
What are the functions of pantothenic acid (B5) to the body?

Answer 1
B5 is involved in the formation of coenzyme A (CoA). CoA is a chemical compound involved in other metabolic

activities in the body and it is responsible for production and digestion of fatty acids. It reduces body cholesterol, low density lipoprotein (LDL)- bad cholesterol, and triglycerides, and it causes rise in good cholesterol called high density cholesterol (HDL). Some studies suggested that it lowers inflammation at early stage, and that it acts as antioxidant.

Question 2
When B5 is low or deficient in the body, how will the body react to it?

Answer 2
Deficiency of vitamin B5 will have the following effects to the body:

Deficiency

Although, it is rare to see a person with vitamin B5 deficiency because it occurs everywhere. However, malnutrition can cause it and a person that have problems digesting vitamin B5 can experience low B5. If B5 is low in the body, it can cause headache, disturbed sleep, fatigue, muscle cramps, numbness or burning sensation in feet and hands, irritability, and restlessness.

Question 3
What is the recommended dietary allowance (RDA) for vitamin B5?

Answer 3
The RDA for vitamin B5 is as follows:

Recommended Dietary Allowance (RDA)

Adults aged 19 years old and above male and female requires only 5 mg per day. Pregnant women, requires 6 mg per day and lactating mother 7 mg per a day
Keeping in mind the lesson about B5 next is about B6.

Pyridoxine - Vitamin B6

It is a naturally occurring water-soluble vitamin in many foods and it is available as supplement as pyridoxal 5' phosphate (PLP). It is a component of coenzyme that is involved in over 100 enzyme activities in the body namely, digestion of fat, carbohydrates, protein, homocysteine, brain function, as well as immune system boosting (7, 8, 47, 66).

Functions

It is a component of coenzyme that is involved in over 100 enzyme activities in the body namely, digestion of fat, carbohydrates, protein, homocysteine, brain function, as well as immune system boosting. Vitamin B6 is good for treating pregnant women who are nauseous, although professional guidance is critical for this. This vitamin may also, lower the risk of cancer (7, 8, 47).

Recommended Dietary Allowance (RDA)

Female aged 14 - 18 requires 1.2 mg, 19 - 50 requires 1.3 mg and 51 years and above needs 1.5 mg per day. Pregnant female requires 1.9 mg and lactating mothers, 2.0 mg per day. Male aged 14-50 requires 1.3 mg per day, and male from 51 years old and above needs 1.7 mg (7, 8, 47).

Deficiency

B6 deficiency, rarely occurs except other B-group vitamins are low essentially folic acid and B12. A prolonged or severe deficiency can result in, microcytic anemia, skin conditions, low immune system, skin conditions, confusion and depression (7, 8, 47).

Conditions that inhibit B6 absorption in the body namely, Alcoholism, inflammations caused by autoimmune disorders example rheumatoid arthritis, autoimmune intestinal disorders namely, ulcers, celiac disease, Crohn's diseases and kidney can result in B6 deficiency (7, 8, 47).

Sources

Plant Sources: banana, avocado, spinach, mango nuts, whole grain bread, cantaloupe, carica papaya, oranges, dark green vegetables, chickpeas, vegetables and fruits.

Animal: Poultry, tuna, salmon, fish, beef liver (7, 8, 47).

Question 1

What are the functions of vitamin B6 (Pyridoxin)?

Answer 1

Vitamin B6 performs several functions and they are listed below:

Functions

It is a component of coenzyme that is involved in over 100 enzyme activities in the body namely, digestion of fat, carbohydrates, protein, homocysteine, brain function, as well as immune system boosting. Good for treating pregnant women who are nauseating, although professional guide is critical for this. It could lower the risk of cancer.

Question 2

What signs will deficiency of vitamin B6 show to the body?

Answer 2

When B6 is low in the body, the following will occur to the body:

Deficiency

B6 deficiency, realty occurs except other B-group vitamins are low essentially folic acid and B12. A prolonged or severe deficiency can result in, microcytic anemia, skin conditions, low immune system, skin conditions, confusion and depression.

Conditions that inhibit B6 absorption in the body namely, Alcoholism, inflammations cause by autoimmune disorders example rheumatoid arthritis, autoimmune intestinal disorders namely, ulcers, celiac disease, Crohn's diseases and kidney can result in B6 deficiency

Question 3
What are the recommended dietary allowance for vitamin B6?

Answer 3
The RDA for B6 is as follows:

Recommended Dietary Allowance (RDA)

Female aged 14-18 requires 1.2 mg, 19-50 requires 1.3 mg and 51 years and above needs 1.5 mg per day. Pregnant female requires 1.9 mg and lactating mothers, 2.0 mg per day. Male aged 14-50 requires 1.3 mg per day, and male from 51 years old and above needs 1.7 mg.

With the lesson about B6 in thoughts next, is about biotin.

Biotin - Vitamin B7

Biotin occurs naturally in some foods and a water-soluble vitamin. It is a co-enzyme that assists enzymes to perform some metabolic processes such as protein, carbohydrates, and lipids digestion. It regulates gene activities, and the signals that the body cells send out to the brain. It is good for the development, growth and hair health. It is good for skin and nail health. It promotes respiration and growth (7, 8, 48).

Functions

It helps enzyme in some metabolic processes such as protein, carbohydrates, and lipids digestion. It regulates gene activities, and signals sent out to the brain by the body cells.

It promotes healthy hair, nails and skin and it prevents hair loss. **Hair loss caused by alopecia is restored with just biotin rich food** (7, 8, 48).

Recommended Dietary Allowance (RDA)

RDA is not available but, there is adequate intake (AI): adult female, male and pregnant mothers, 30 mg per day is suggested and 35 mg advised fro lactating mothers per day (7, 8, 48).

Deficiency

Hair loss, nail and skin problems. Biotin functions mentioned above can be affected when it is deficient in the body, It will result in biotin deficiency.

It will result into scaly skin rashes around mouth, nose and eyes, brittle nails, and thin hair. Alcoholism, and raw egg consumption can cause biotin deficiency. Raw egg contains avidin, which clings or binds to biotin and make it unavailable for absorption. Avidin in raw egg is denatured or weakened after cooking (7, 8, 48).

Sources

Plants: Sweet potatoes, yam, nuts, seeds, and avocado. Animals: Egg, pork, fish, salmon, and beef liver (7, 8, 48).

Question 1
What are the recommended dietary allowance (RDA) for biotin?

Answer 1
Biotin has no RDA but, there is adequate intake (AI): adult female, male and pregnant mothers, 30 mg per day is suggested and 35 mg advised for lactating mothers per day.

Question 2
How will deficiency of biotin manifest in the body?

Answer 2
When biotin is too low in the body the it will manifest in these forms:

Deficiency

Hair loss, nail and skin problems. Biotin functions mentioned above can be affected when it is deficient in the body, It will result in biotin deficiency.

It will cause scaly skin rashes around mouth, nose and eyes, brittle nails, and thin hair. Alcoholism, and raw egg consumption can cause biotin deficiency.

Question 3

What are the sources of vitamin B7?

Answer 3

Biotin can be obtained from plants and animals sources:

Sources

Plants: Sweet potatoes, yam, nuts, seeds, and avocado. **Animals**: Egg, pork, fish, salmon, and beef liver.

Keeping in mind the lesson about biotin next, is about B9.

Folate: Folic Acid - Vitamin B9

Folate is a naturally occurring water-soluble vitamin in many foods from plant and animal alike. There is also folate supplement - folic acid, which has better absorption, 85% absorption than natural folic acid, which only 50% of it is absorbed. It is involved in RNA and DNA formation, and protein metabolism (7, 8, 49). It has a capacity to break down a harmful amino acid in the body called homocysteine. Essential for the formation of healthy red blood cells, and during rapid growth in children, pregnancy and development of the fetus (7, 8, 49).

Function

It is involved in RNA and DNA formation, and protein metabolism. It has a capacity to break down a harmful amino acid in the body called homocysteine. Essential for the formation of healthy red blood cells, and during rapid growth in children, pregnancy and development of the fetus ((7, 8, 49).

Recommended Dietary Allowance (RDA)

Measured in microgram (ug) dietary folate equivalents (DFE). Male and female aged 19 years old and above require 400 mcg DFE. Lactating mother, 500 mcg, and pregnant mother requires 600 mcg daily. Please, note that alcohol hinders folate absorption (7, 8, 49).

Deficiency

Deficiency of folate is a rare occurrence. Deficiency of folate is caused by alcoholism, pregnancy, and intestinal surgeries or digestive disorders that cause food malabsorption. Also persons with a genetic variant called MTHFR cannot digest folate (7, 8, 49).

Sources

Folate occurs widely in nature in plant and animal food sources alike.

Plant sources: parboiled brown rice, pasta, grain food, cereals, dark green leafy vegetables, example, green tete, fluted pumpkin leaves, bitter leaves, kale, spinach, turnip greens, romaine lettuce, asparagus, broccoli, Brussels sprout, beans, peanut, sunflower seeds, while grains and fresh fruits, and faith juices.

Animal: Liver, egg, seafood, fortified foods and supplements (7, 8, 49).

Question 1
What are sources of folic acid (B9)?

Answer 1
These are sources of B9:

Sources

Folate occurs widely in nature in plant and animal food sources alike.

Plant sources: parboiled brown rice, pasta, grain food, cereals, dark green leafy vegetables, example, green tete, fluted pumpkin leaves, bitter leaves, kale, spinach, turnip greens, romaine lettuce, asparagus, broccoli, Brussels sprout, beans, peanut, sunflower seeds, while grains and fresh fruits, and faith juices.

Animal: Liver, egg, seafood, fortified foods and supplements.

Question 2
When B9 is deficient in the body, how does the body react?

Answer 2
Deficiency of B9 will manifest in the body in the following ways:

Deficiency

Deficiency of folate is a rare occurrence. Deficiency of folate is caused by alcoholism, pregnancy, and intestinal surgeries or digestive disorders that cause food malabsorption. Also persons with a genetic variant called MTHFR cannot digest folate.

Question 3
What are the recommended dietary allowance (RDA) for B9?

Answer 3
The RDA for B9 are as follows:

Recommended Dietary Allowance (RDA)

B9 is measured in microgram (ug) dietary folate equivalents (DFE). Male and female aged 19 years old and above require 400 mcg, DFE. Lactating mother, 500 mcg, and pregnant mother requires 600 mcg daily. Please, note that alcohol hinders folate absorption.

Question 4
What are the functions of B9 to the body?

Answer 4
Folate performs the following functions to the body:

Function

It is involved in RNA and DNA formation, and protein metabolism. It has a capacity to break down a harmful amino acid in the body called homocysteine. It is essential for the formation of healthy red blood cells, and during rapid growth in children, pregnancy and development of the fetus.

With the lesson about B9 in mind next, is about B12.

Cobalamin - Vitamin B12

Cobalamin is a water-soluble vitamin that occur naturally in animal foods only. It can be used to fortify food and it is available as supplement. It is a major factor in the brain and nerve cells formation, as well as DNA and red blood cells formation. B12 naturally binds to protein cells. After the consumption of protein that contains B12, the hydrochloric acid (HCL) involved in protein digestion dislodges or separates it from the protein to assume its free state in a form that the body can absorb it (7, 8, 50). Unlike the naturally occurring B12, which binds to protein and needs HCL to separate it from protein before the body can utilize it; foods fortified with B12 and B12 supplements contains B12 that is in free state - ready for the body to use it. It is necessary to note that **B12 supplement usually comes in doses higher than the recommended dietary allowance (RDA) because not all will be absorbed** in the body (7, 8, 50). Also, person not having enough intrinsic factor - suffering from pernicious anemia, which hinders the function of intrinsic also affects B12 cell absorption. Pernicious anemia is an autoimmune disease that destroys gut cells thereby inhibiting B12 absorption. In this case high dose of B12 cannot fix it, may be B12 injection can (7, 8, 50).

Function

It is a major factor in brain and nerve cells formation, as well as DNA and red blood cells formation (7, 8, 50).

Deficiency

B12 deficiency, those who avoid poultry, meat, fish and dairy products are at risk of B12 deficiency. Fifteen percent (15%) of United States general population are estimated to be deficient in vitamin B12. Also, blood analysis or test in some cases do not accurately measure the level of B12 in the body (7, 8, 50). Thus, analysts should focus on determining the concentration of homocysteine, methylmalonic acid, and protein break down products because when their concentrations in the blood are high, it is a clear sign that vitamin B12 is deficient in the blood of that person (7, 8, 50).

Other factors that Cause B12 Deficiency are:

When people avoid animal food or products, absence of intrinsic fact or presence of pernicious anemia, and low stomach acid or medications that cause low stomach acid, surgery on the intestine and digestive disorders cause malabsorption of cobalamin (B12) (7, 8, 50).

Other signs of B12 deficiency are: Seizures, depression, dementia, memory loss, confusion, fatigue, weakness, nerve damage that cause numbness, and cause legs and hands to tingle (7, 8, 50).

Recommended Dietary Allowance (RDA)

Female and male aged 14 years and above requires 2.4 microgram (mcg) per a day. Pregnant woman requires 2.6 mcg and lactating mother's require 2.8 mcg per day (7, 8, 50).

Sources

Source are only from animal food and animal food products only namely, meat, poultry, fish, egg, sea foods, milk, and lean meat (7, 8, 50).

Question 1

What are the recommended dietary allowance (RDA) for B12?

Answer 1
The RDA for B12 (cobalamin) are:

Recommended Dietary Allowance (RDA)

Female and male aged 14 years and above requires 2.4 microgram (mcg) per a day. Pregnant woman requires 2.6 mcg and lactating mother's require 2.8 mcg per day (7, 8, 50).

Question 2
What are the sources of B12?

Answer 2

Sources

The sources are from animal food and animal food products only namely, meat, poultry, fish, egg, sea foods, milk, and lean meat.

Question 3
How will low B12 manifest in the body?

Answer 3
When B12 is too low in the body it will result into:

Deficiency

Persons that avoid poultry, meat, fish and dairy products are at risk of B12 deficiency. Fifteen percent (15%) of United States general population are estimated to be deficient in vitamin B12. Also, blood analysis or test in some cases do not accurately measure the level of B12 in the body (7, 8, 50). Thus, analysts should focus on determining the concentration of homocysteine, methylmalonic acid, and protein break down products because when their concentrations in the blood are high, it is an indication that vitamin B12 is deficient in that person.

Other signs of B12 deficiency are:Seizures, depression, dementia, memory loss, confusion, fatigue, weakness, nerve damage that cause numbness, and cause legs and hands to tingle

Question 4
Aside, abstinence from animal food, what other factors can cause B12 deficiency?

Answer 4
Other factors that Cause B12 Deficiency outside animal products abstinence are:
Absence of intrinsic fact or presence of pernicious anemia, and low stomach acid or medications that cause low stomach acid, surgery on the intestine and digestive disorders that cause malabsorption of cobalamin (B12).

Question 5
What are the functions of B12 to the body?

Answer 5
Cobalamin performs critical functions to the body and they are listed as:

Function

It is a major factor needed in the brain and nerve cells formation. It is essential for DNA and red blood cells formation.

With the lesson about B12 in thoughts next, it may interest you to read about how B-group vitamins emerged from B-complex and B2-complex.

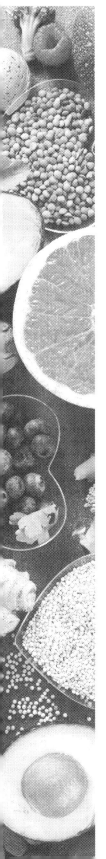

Chapter 8

Discovery of B-group Vitamins: B2 (Riboflavin) Emerges From B Complex

When liver, yeasts and rice bran were autoclaved and thiamin-free extract from them fed to rat, that were also given thiamin supplement, the rat were able to grow. B complex is a growth factor, water-soluble and stable at high temperature (heat stable). Also, yellow-green fluorescence found in the extract supported growth, and the level of growth was proportional to the intensity of the fluorescence (7, 8). The same growth factor called fluorescence was isolated from egg as *ovoflavin*, from the whey protein of milk as *lactoflavin*. These growth factor then became *flavins*, and for the fact that these flavins consist of rinotyl (ribos-like) portion, they came up with a general name for the growth factor as riboflavin, and that becomes the vitamin B2. It is also acting as a metabolite- coenzyme necessary for metabolic processes (7; 8).

Question 1
A growth factor found in Yeast, rice bran, egg (ovoflavin), whey milk protein (lactoflavin), which was flavin and also act as coenzyme metabolite is called what?

Answer 1
It is called riboflavin- vitamin B2 because it contains flavin, and it is ribos-like.

Question 2
Riboflavin emerged from which B group vitamins?

Answer 2
It emerged from B complex.

Niacin Emerges from B2 Complex

A filtrate of B Complex from Fuller's Earth gave birth to anti pellagra (P-P) factor, which prevented canine-black tongue. This anti pellagra and anti black tongue P-P factor then emerged as nicotinamide and nicotinic acid, which is now known as niacin (B3) (7).

Question 1
What is the anti-pellagra and anti-black tongue obtained from the filtrate of B2 complex from Fuller's Earth is called?

Answer1
It is called niacin (B3) or nicotinamide or nicotinic acid. Keeping in mind the lesson about how niacin emerged from B2 complex next, is a lesson about emergence of B6 from B2 complex.
Keeping in mind the lesson about how niacin emerged from B2 complex, next, is a lesson about emergence of B6 from B2 complex.

Pyridoxin(B6) Emerges from B2 Complex

Anonymous relationship between growth-factor (flourescence) and growth promoting led to more studies on B complex. Since the promotion of fluorescence and the growth promoted was not proportionately correlated as earlier suggested, the non-florescence extract was added to fluorescence and it prevented dermatitis in rat (adermin), which was not the same as lesion diseases caused by deficiency of riboflavin (B2). This third growth-factor was named pyridoxine-vitamin B6 with chemical structure, 3-hydroxy-4,5-bis (hydroxymethyl)-2-methylpyridinr (7).

Question 1
What was the growth promoting factor, which is not growth-factor-fluorescence, but when added to growth-factor-fluorescence prevented dermatitis in rat called?

Answer 1: It is called non-fluorescence extract.

Question 2
What is the third growth-factor that emerged when fluorescence and non-fluorescence extract that prevented dermatitis in rat were added together?

Answer 2: It is called pantothenic acid- vitamin B5, it is also called anti-dermatitis factor.

With the lesson about emergence of pantothenic acid from B2 complex in mid, next, is about emergence of vitamin B7 (biotin) from bios.

Pantothenic Acid Emerges from B2 Complex

Further investigation on B2 complex discovered that there is yet another growth factor component of B2 complex, which its deficiency caused a diseases in chicken that resembles pellagra. The name of the disease is lesion and aqueous extract of liver and yeast prevented the diseases from occurring (7, 8). The growth factor was a residue or filtrate obtained after filtering B2 complex through the *Fuller's Earth*, which was stable at high temperature. This growth factor occurs widely in varieties of plants and animals found everywhere; hence the name, pantothenic acid. Pantothenic acid (vitamin B5) was identified as anti dermatitis factor because it was able to inhibit dermatitis and poor feather in chicken, and it is a required growth factor for bacterial and yeasts (saccharomyces cerevisiae) as well as chicken (7, 8). B2 emerged from B complex, and B3, B6, and B5 emerged from B2 complex.

Question 1
The fourth growth factor that emerged from vitamin B2 Complex obtained from residue after filtering B2 complex through Fuller's Earth, stable at high temperature found everywhere, which prevented dermatitis and poor feather growth in chicken, and it is a required growth factor for chicken, yeast and bacterial is called what?

Answer 1
It is called pantothenic acid- vitamin B5, it is also called anti-dermatitis factor.
With the lesson about emergence of pantothenic acid from B2 complex in mid next, is about emergence of vitamin B7 (biotin) from bios

Biotin (vitamin B7) emerges from Bios

Yet another growth factor emerged from yeast, which was identified as bios. More investigations on yeast led to the discovery of another growth fact, which promotes respiration and growth in humans and animals. It is good for the development, growth and maintenance of healthy hair in humans and lower animals. The newly revealed growth factor was found to be a co-enzyme. It was named **coenzyme R**, which is also called *Rhizobium trifolii*.

The newly discovered growth factor prevented skin hair loss in rats and lesion caused by feeding rats with raw egg white (7, 8). A growth factor (vitamin H) was not only obtained from yeast, it was also isolated from egg yolk, and a preparation made from the liver. The growth factor from egg yoke and the preparation made from the liver was vitamin H, which is biotin and it prevented rats from skin hair loss and lesion that they developed when they were fed with raw egg white. The factor was named biotin. It is neither vitamins A, C, D, E, nor vitamin K. It is is good for skin, nail, and hair health in humans, and hair loss caused by alopecia can be restored fully with just biotin rich food (7, 8, 48)

Please, NOTE that avidin from raw or uncooked egg white can prevent or inhibit biotin absorption but when cooked, avidin inhibiting power is lost to cooking (7, 21, 43).

Question 1

A growth factor isolated from egg yoke, which is similar from preparation made from the liver that prevented skin hair loss and lesion of rat, which is not vitamins A, C, D, E and K is called what?

Answer 1

It is vitamin H, also called biotin or B7

Question 2

What content of egg white prevents biotin absorption when uncooked?

Answer 2

Avidin of raw or uncooked egg white prevents biotin from absorption in the body but, when cooked it does not prevent its absorption.

With the lesson about the emergence of biotin from bios next is about vitamin C.

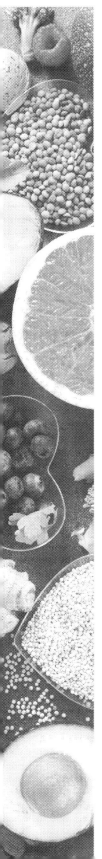

Chapter 9

Water-Soluble: Vitamin C: Ascorbic Acid

In the 1070s, a researcher called Linus Pauling a two-time Nobel Laureate winner and champion of vitamin C promoted that the increase of intake of orange juice or Vitamin C tablet is necessary to overcome cold and many diseases including chronic diseases and recommended 12-24 oranges per day to achieve that. Vitamin C is heat sensitive and water soluble thus, exposure to heat and water will cause its loss (7, 8). It is potent against infectious diseases, wound healing, preventing and healing scurvy, and a powerful antioxidant that neutralizes free radicals that are harmful to the human body. Vitamin C is essential for collagen formation. Collagen is a cell fibre in the human tissue that is located in various parts of the body system namely, in the immune system, bone, cartilage, blood, and nerves (7, 8).

Vitamin C was discovered to be capable of reducing a dye, 2,6-dichloroindophenol; however, when the reducing function of vitamin C was bioassayed (investigated), the reducing function of vitamin C assayed with reagent correlated with antiscorbutic function sometimes but, not all the times that it was tested. The cause of irregular correlation of vitamin C in some cases was due to reverse oxidation that occurs with vitamin C (7, 8). Vitamin C was isolated from adrenal cortex, cabbage and citrus juice. It was used to prevent and treat scurvy (7, 8). Thus there were two forms of vitamin C namely, reduced vitamin C and oxidized vitamin C. It is worthy of note that both reduced and oxidized vitamin C were able to perform the antiscorbutic function. And it was later established that the antiscorbutic factor is identical to ascorbic acid (hexuronic acid) (7, 8).

Recommended Daily Allowance (RDA) for Vitamin C

For male adults 19 years and above, 90 mg per day is recommended, and female aged 18 years and above, 75 mg daily. Pregnant women and lactating mothers a range of 85-120 mg per day is recommended. Since smoking depletes vitamin C level significantly, smokers are recommended to take extra 35 mg daily to protect (16, 22).

Upper Limit consumption of vitamin C is 2000 my per day. Above the upper limit can be toxic to the body (16, 22)

Functions

It is potent against infectious diseases as a strong immune system booster, and against chronic diseases as a powerful antioxidant. It promotes wound healing, prevents and heals scurvy, and it is a powerful antioxidant that neutralizes harmful free radicals in the body. Vitamin C is essential for collagen formation. Collagen is a cell fibre in the human tissue that is located in various parts of the body system namely, in the immune system, bone, cartilage, blood, and nerves (16, 22). It is used to reduce excess iron in the body.

Deficiency

Severe deficiency of vitamin C results in the disease of the mouth called scurvy, loss of collagen and weakness of connective tissues. It causes ruptures of the blood vessels that result in spots, bruising and bleeding. Vitamin C deficiency causes swelling of the gum, bleeding, and loss of teeth. It delays the healing time of wound, hair loss and malaise (general feeling of discomfort or ill), and fatigue (16, 22).

Question 1
Why was vitamin C not capable of performing reducing function always?

Answer 1
Because vitamin C occurs in two forms the reduced and oxidized forms, when it is in oxidized form it cannot perform its reducing function but when it is in reduced vitamin C form, it is able to perform its reducing function.

Question 2
Are reduced and oxidized vitamin C capable of performing antiscorbutic function?

Answer 2
Yes, they are

Table 1. Recommended Dietary Allowance for Vitamins

Vitamins	Unit	Upper Limit (UL) PRI or AI EU	Upper Limit (UL) PRI or AI US	Upper Limit (UL) Japan	EAR US AI	RDA or AI US Highest	PRI or AI EU
Vitamin E	mg	300	1000	650-900	12	15	13
Vitamin B1	mg	ND	ND	ND	1	1.2	0.1mg/MJ
Vitamin B2- Riboflavin	mg	ND	ND	ND	1.1	1.3	2
Vitamin B3-Niacin	mg	10	35	60-85	12	16	1.6mg/MJ
Vitamin B5- Pantothenic acid	mg	ND	ND	ND	NE	5	7
Vitamin B6- Pyridoxin	mg	25	100	40-60	1.1	1.3	1.8
Biotin B7	ug	ND	ND	ND	NE	30	45
Folate B9	ug	1000	1000	900-1000	320	400	600
Cyanocobalamin B12	ug	ND	ND	ND	2	2.4	5

(21).

AI US and EFSA Adequate Intake; EARs and RDAs are used to estimate limits when no sufficient data is established for nutrient to be AI.

Definition of terms

Upper limit (UL): Tolerable upper level of intake

RDA: Recommended daily Allowance, US

AI: Adequate intake

ND: Not determined

NE: EARs not estimated

PRI: Population reference intake, it is European Union equivalent of US RDA

MJ: Mega joule: 239 of food calories

With the lesson about vitamins C in thoughts next, is about the clarifications of myths and facts in nutrition and health.

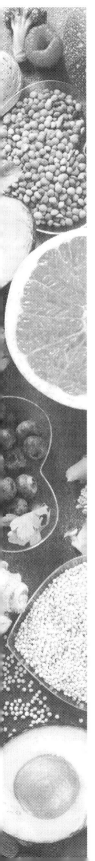

Chapter 10

Clarification of Myth and facts about Vitamins

Here are facts about vitamins and their health functions to the body. In the past a disease called beriberi was feared to be an infectious disease. This was wrong. Beriberi is not infectious disease, it is a disease developed for lack of eating B-group vitamins, which naturally occurs predominantly in cereals. In similar vein scurvy was mistreated as a contagious disease but, it was not a contagious disease rather, it is a disease that usually occurs when people eat food that lacks vitamin C (ascorbic acid) (7) for a long time.

Vitamin A was named "**a growth factor**": the meaning of this phrase is that it is essential for growth. Fetus, infants, and animals that were deficient in vitamin A experienced stunted growth or no growth. Deficiency of vitamin A affects the vision as well and cause night blindness and xerophthalmia, night blindness, and xerophthalmia (defect of cornea and conjunctiva of the eye caused by lack of vitamin A) (7, 8, 29, 30, 31).

When cod liver oil, which is a rich source of vitamin A was abetted (intentionally subjected to heat for the purpose of changing it to vitamin D) and heated, the oil lost its vitamin A value, and rather obtained vitamin D status instead because, when it was fed to the animals, the animals were not protected from xerophthalmia (extreme case of conjunctivitis) but, were protected from rachitic (rickets) (7, 8). Rickets is a bone disease caused by deficiency of vitamin D that affect the legs and cause it to bend.

Thus, vitamin A is said to be antixerophthalmia and vitamin D antirachitic- preventing rickets. Beta carotene is a precursor of vitamin A. This means that beta-carotene when consumed, it is easily convert to vitamin A to supply the body vitamin A. In similar vein an amino acid called tryptophan is a provitamin B3 (niacin). When tryptophan is consumed and there is no niacin in the body, tryptophan can be used by the body to produce niacin.

Prior to this study this author believed that vitamin D can only be obtained through exposure of uncovered skin to the sun, and many people in the tropics share in this believe; however, through this study, this author came to a conviction that vitamin D can enter human and animal bodies through other means. Other than exposure to direct sun, humans and animals can obtain vitamin D through food exposed to the sun and ultraviolet irradiation a person or animals or food given to them. Ultraviolet irradiation of animals or food fed to animals brought cure for rickets or rachitic. Vitamin D comes in two forms called vitamers namely, D2 and D3.

It is important to note that, whether vitamin D was synthesized by exposure to sunshine, ingested orally through supplements, or synthesized by artificial means it is not absorbed in the body until it is metabolized (digested) by metabolic enzymes into a form that the body can absorb, which is called metabolites. Additionally, vitamin D is called a steroid hormone, making it to act as a vitamin as well as a hormone. Researchers are investigating other essential functions of vitamin D to the body (7, 8).

B-group vitamins are sensitive to heat. Heat denatures some of them. Because yeast is good source of B-group vitamins, it was used to prevent Beriberi and pellagra making B group vitamins or yeast anti neuritis ("A-N" or anti-beriberi) and anti-pellagra ("P-P"-pellagra preventive). Pellagra is caused by lack or deficiency of vitamin B3 (Niacin). Symptoms of niacin deficiency are sore in the mouth, diarrhoea, dermatitis, and dementia. However, when it was denatured by heat it could still prevent dermatitis. The anti neuritis -"A-N" and anti-pellagra-"P-P" later became vitamins B1 and B2 (7, 8, 39). There are several factors about vitamin B2. Examples, some are stable at high temperatures, and some are unstable and are destroyed by heat, and some perform different functions to the body and to different animals. For these reasons a name B complex was given to it because:

It prevented pellagra in human, monkeys, pigs, dogs, and rat, it is a growth factor for rat and prevented dermatitis in chicken.

With the lesson about clarifications of myths and facts in nutrition and health in thoughts next, is about an overview of micronutrients.

Question 1

How did the name B complex come about?

Answer 1

Because, vitamin B has vitamers, namely, vitamins B1-12. Some are unstable at high temperature, some are stable at high temperature. Some prevent beriberi (anti neuritis (A-N), and some are anti-pellagra ("P-P" - preventing pellagra). When denatured by heat it prevents dermatitis. It prevents pellagra in human, monkey, pig, dog and rat. It is a growth factor for rat and it prevents dermatitis in chicken.

With the lesson about clarifications of myths and facts in nutrition and health in thoughts, next, is about an overview of micronutrients.

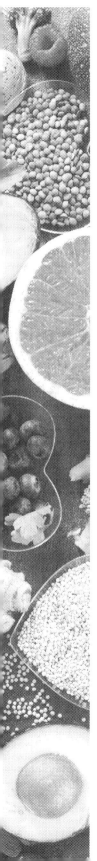

Chapter 11

Micronutrients Overview

Before going into a discussion about specific minerals, lets have a general discussion about minerals and trace elements because they play essential roles in human nutrition and well being. They are also called elements. There are about 112 elements, out of these, only 21 are required in human nutrition (nutriture). Eleven of them are needed in relatively bigger quantity than the rest of nine. The eleven are calcium, sodium, magnesium, hydrogen, carbon, oxygen, nitrogen, potassium, phosphorus, chlorine and sulphur (7, 8, 51, 52, 53, 54, 55).

These elements form the essential building blocks of the nucleic acid, lipids, protein, and carbohydrates, and play critical role of intracellular and extracellular electrolytes. It is worthy of note that **only magnesium, calcium**, and **phosphorus** out of 11 essential elements have recommended dietary allowances (RDAs). The fact is that some of the rest occur predominantly in all parts of the body as a major component of the body cells, and the task of determining their RDAs could be cumbersome and yet with little value. There is no RDAs for Oxygen, sulphurs and carbon. Oxygen and hydrogen are components of water (7, 8, 51, 52, 53, 55).

There are nine essential trace elements namely, iron, manganese, iodine, zinc, selenium, molybdenum, flourine, chromium, copper. It is important to note that cobalt is not essential trace element; however, it is an essential part of vitamin B12. The RDAs, or Estimated Safe Adequate and Daily Intakes (ESADDIs) for chromium, copper, fluoride, manganese, and molybdenum, as well as iron, zinc, selenium, and iodine are generally low; however, that of iron, zinc, iodine, and selenium is of higher value. Calcium, magnesium, and phosphorus are relatively required in the body in a larger quantity compared with the trace elements hence, they are NOT regarded as trace elements 7, 8, 51, 52, 53, 55).

Trace elements are required in the body in trace amount ranging from tens of micrograms (ug) to tens of milligrams (mg). As much as 40% of the global population faces deficiency in one or more trace element. About 2 billion are lacking iron, 1.5 billion are lacking iodine, 5.6 billion for zinc; then, selenium and copper 7, 8, 51, 52, 53, 55).

Question 1
What are three out of 11 essential elements that have recommended dietary allowance?
Answer: They Magnesium, Calcium and Phosphorus.

Question 2
What are nine essential trace elements?

Answer: They are iron, manganese, iodine, zinc, selenium, molybdenum, flourine, chromium, copper.

Factors Affecting Microminerals Nutriture (Availability and Absorption)

While trace elements or micronutrients are required in the body in trace amount to perform specific metabolic functions, it is worthy of note that some variables or factors influence elements' availability and function in the body. The variables are, interaction between them and other micronutrients, dose-response effect, chelation, oxidation state, binding to macronutrients, and enzyme, bioavailability, and immutability (7, 8, 51, 52, 53, 55).

Interaction

Interactions between elements and other nutrients and even enzymes can affect availability and function of the elements in the body. Here are a few examples, people consuming high doses of zinc for long period of time owing to deficiency of copper can cause anemia. It is yet not clear whether daily consumption of 15-25 mg can compromise bio availability of copper-can cause copper deficiency. Selenium reduces mercury toxicity (7, 8, 51, 52, 53, 55).

Presence of tiny initial dose of cadmium can protect the body against toxicity of large dose of cadmium and mercury through its initiation of synthesis and storage of of low weight protein called metallothioneins-amino acid rich in sulphur in the liver and kidneys and this amino acid compound is capable of binding with subsequent cadmium and mercury to reduce their toxic effect (7, 8, 51, 52, 53, 55).

High calcium and magnesium obtained from diet has positive effect at inhibiting lead absorption in the gastrointestine, Calcium also, affects the absorption of iron, zinc, and molybdenum, and it can lower the retention of copper. A list of examples of elements interaction that stand in the way for elements absorption or metabolic functions is continuous. It is important to note that not knowing exact amount of some of this elements in the body stands a chance of compromising its availability, absorption and function thus, it may be necessary to know them (7, 8, 51, 52, 53, 55).

Dose-Response Effect

It is necessary to evaluate dose-response effect in determining element level in the body. Low level or deficiency can results in diseases since deficiencies are associated with diseases but, excess intake can be toxic to the body, and it can lead to death in some situations example zinc toxicity can lead to death. Cadmium is essential for rat growth but, excess is toxic to rat's kidney (7, 8, 51, 52, 53, 55).

Oxidation State

An oxidation state of trace elements affects its availability, absorption and function. For example, chromium when in dietary form with oxidation state of +3, even at high concentration, is essential and can be tolerated in the body; but, when it is +6 oxidation state it is no longer essential and it becomes toxic (7, 8, 51, 52, 53, 55). Also, when chromate gets into the body through inhalation, it is highly carcinogenic but when it gets into the body through cellular and intracellular processes, it is not but, what is toxic is the conversion of chromate with oxidation state of +6 to oxidation state of +3. Zinc has one oxidative state +2 (7, 8, 51, 52, 53, 55).

Enzymes and Hormones

Trace metal elements are significantly essential elements because they interact and perform joint function with hormones and enzymes. Many enzymes contain at least one essential trace element. For example one molecule of copper-transporting protein named ceruloplasmin contains 8 atoms of copper. Other enzymes containing copper are, cytochrome-c-oxidase, lysyl oxidase, tryosinase, and cytosolic superoxide dismutase (7, 8, 51, 52, 53, 55).

Also, metalloenzymes namely, alkaline phosphatase, alcohol dehydrogenase, carbonic anhydrase, RNA polymerase, and ALA dehydratase, contains a metal called zinc. And the presence and function of zinc in these and many other enzymes accounts for many adverse effect that the body experience in zinc deficient animal. It affects growth as well as the immune system. Some enzymes also consist of two elements example cytosolic superoxide dismutase, which consists of copper and zinc. ALA dehydratase is also called Delta-aminolevulinic acid dehydratase or aminolevulinate dehydratase (7, 8, 51, 52, 53, 55).

Other elements found in enzymes are selenium found in glutathione peroxidase, mitochondrial superoxide dismutase containing manganese, and Xanthine oxidase consisting of molybdenum.

Trace element activity in hormone function is exemplified by iodine function in thyroid hormone (7, 8, 51, 52, 53, 55).

Chelating

Presence of a chelating agent can interfere with trace element availability. When an agent is chelating. It means that there is a presence of ligand or molecule that can bind with transition metals namely, copper, chromium, iron, molybdenum, and manganese. The bond can be more than one such as, bidentate (2), terdentate (3), quadridentate (4), quintuidentate (5) or multi dentate, the bonds can be formed with sulphur, oxygen, and nitrogen atoms, between chelating agent and the trace metals.

Macromolecules and enzymes could become chelating especially, if they have oxygen, nitrogen, and sulphur atoms. Medicines implicated are, ethambutol, penicilliamine, and ethylenediamine-tetra acetate (EDTA), physicians prescribing these medications need to factor that into consideration (7, 8, 51, 52, 53, 55).

Chelating medicine namely penicillamine, which is a bidentate molecule is effective for excess coper excretion from organ such as that caused by Wilson diseases and lead poisoning. This critical action results in zinc excretion, which causes deficiency of zinc, very important to note (7, 8, 51, 52, 53, 55).

Immutability

Trace elements are immutable-never changing; however, they can become oxidized and their position in the bonding can shift. It is hard for its level or concentration to change. In-vitro change may occur to them but external items can alter the quantity of trace elements. Care must be taken with sampling tools to avoid external contamination. Example rubber stopper is capable of contaminating blood sample with zinc (7, 8, 51, 52, 53, 55).

Bioavailability

A situation where zinc quantity in food is enough but if a person consumes food that contains phytate, this can cause deficiency of zinc because phytate interferes with zinc absorption in the intestine. Zinc can also interact with vitamin C, copper, and iron, and this can affect bioavailability of those elements and vitamin C (7, 8, 51, 52, 53, 55).

Absorption and Excretion

Absorption and excretion problems can also, cause deficiency of trace-elements. When excess iron accumulates in the organ by a process called hemochromatosis, it results in organ's inability to control certain elements such as iron, preventing its absorption and causing toxicity.

Another example is manganese toxicity occurring as a result of defective or ineffective biliary excretion of the liver causing either serious manganese toxicity or fatality (death). These conditions including Wilson disease, which generate situations of high metal accumulation in the organs, which are toxic to the cells and cause cell damage (7, 8, 51, 52, 53, 55).

Cause and Effect

When trace elements are altered, it can generate life-threatening conditions. A severe deficiency of zinc can cause severe impairment of the immune system function. Also, there are diseases and conditions that can negatively affect metabolism of trace elements (7, 8, 51, 52, 53, 55). A typical example is that of copper metabolism, which affect the amount of copper circulated to the body cells, and this negative outcome affects the ability to monitor body responses to chemotherapy. Also, during pregnancy, the metabolism of zinc, iron, and copper is altered (7, 8, 51, 52, 53, 55). When iron is deficient in pregnancy, copper levels rises in mother's liver and placenta causing reduction of copper and rise of zinc in the fetus' liver (69).

Diseases Treatment

It is worthy of note that treatment of certain disease can cause elements' deficiency in the body. Tuberculosis treatment drug called Ethambutol, which is a chelating agent interacts with zinc to decrease sharpness of vision-blurred vision. Also treating Wilson disease with penicillamine causes the body to manifest zinc and copper deficiency. Additionally patients placed on total parenteral nutrition (TPN) often experience deficiencies of trace elements if the TPN is low in the elements (7, 8, 51, 52, 53, 55). TPN is an act of infusing a special form of food usually in liquid form into the body through the vein.

Effects of Pharmacology

In certain conditions, high dose of trace elements can have beneficial or negative (adverse) effects, especially when there is no deficiency experience. For example, high dose of zinc is useful in treating common cold, and an effective treatment of Wilson's disease. Aspirin is another typical example, it is efficient in the treatment of inflammation and pain for a short period. And it's daily low dose consumption is effective in preventing heart attack (7, 8, 51, 52, 53, 55).

Question

What are the factors that affects micronutrient nuriture or availability for body cell use?

There are 11 factors that affect availability of micronutrients or its nuriture to the body. They are:

i. Interactions - with other elements or compounds or enzyme making it unavailable or low in concentration.

ii. Dose-response - when the concentration of micronutrient is too low to provide the necessary nuriture to the body or too high when it becomes toxic to the body

iii. Oxidation - when micro mineral is oxidized, it affects its absorption, utilization and function Example, chromium when in dietary form with oxidation state of +3, even at high concentration, is essential and can be tolerated in the body; but, when it is +6 oxidation state, it is no longer essential and it becomes toxic.

iv. Enzymes and hormones - many trace elements interact and perform joint function with hormones and enzymes. Many enzymes contain at least one essential trace element. For example one molecule of copper-transporting protein named ceruloplasmin contains 8 atoms of copper. These interactions can cause low concentrations or high concentrations which can hinder availability, absorption, utilization and function.

v. Chelating - Presence of a chelating agent can interfere with trace element availability. When an agent is chelating, it means that there is a presence of a ligand or molecule that can bind with transition metals, namely, copper, chromium, iron, molybdenum, and manganese.

vi. Immutability - Trace elements are immutable-never changing; however, they can become oxidized. Also, their position in the bonding can shift. It is hard for its level or concentration to change.

vii. Bioavailability - A situation where zinc quantity in food is enough, if the person consumes food that contains phytate, this can yet cause deficiency of zinc because it interferes with zinc absorption in the intestine. Zinc can also interact with vitamin C, copper, and iron, and this can affect bioavailability of those elements and vitamin C.

viii. Absorption and Excretion - Absorption and excretion problems can also, cause deficiency of trace-elements. When excess iron accumulates in the organ by a process called hemochromatosis, it results in organ's inability to control certain elements such as iron, preventing its absorption and toxicity. Another example is manganese toxicity occurring as a result of defective or ineffective biliary excretion of the liver causing either serious manganese toxicity or fatality (death).

ix. Diseases treatment - Treatment of certain disease can cause elements' deficiency in the body. Tuberculosis treatment drug called Ethambutol, which is a chelating agent interacts with zinc to decrease sharpness of vision causing blurred vision. Also treating Wilson disease with penicillamine causes the body to manifest zinc and copper deficiency.

x. Cause and Effect: Severe deficiencies of trace elements can cause life-threatening diseases. Example severe deficiency of zinc can result in the impairment of immunity functions. Also, there are diseases and conditions that can negatively affect metabolism of trace elements. A typical example is that of copper metabolism, which affect the amount of copper circulated to the body cells, and this negative outcome affects the ability to monitor body responses to chemotherapy. Also, during pregnancy, the metabolism of zinc, iron, and copper is altered.

xi. Pharmacological effect - high dose of trace elements can have beneficial or negative (adverse) effects, especially when there is no deficiency experience. For example, high dose of zinc is useful in treating common cold, and an effective treatment of Wilson's disease. Aspirin is another typical example, it is efficient in the treatment of inflammation and pain for a short period. And it's daily low dose consumption is effective in preventing heart attack. Determining the body concentration of trace element is a necessary guide to determine the right quantity or dose for a person (7, 8, 51, 52, 53, 55).

Please, not that except zinc that has a question, there will be no further questions following each lessons starting from sulfur to the end. It is amounting to repetitions and taking up spaces. I leave the questions up to the teachers and readers to use the question patterns above or other patterns to formulate questions for the lessons.

With the knowledge of micronutrients overview and the knowledge of conditions that affect availability and absorption in mind, next, let's learn about specific micronutrients nuriture, essentiality, and terms used to describe nutritional effect.

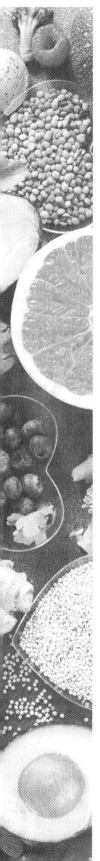

Chapter 12

Micronutrient: Minerals Nuriture

Mineral is described as inorganic elements required essentially for various life functions by human beings and organism (16, 21). About 96% of the human body structure consist of oxygen, carbon, nitrogen, and hydrogen yet, non of those is counted as main body nutrient. Trace or minor elements and vitamins constitute the rest (16, 21). Some mineral elements have been implicated as having capacity to prevent diseases, enhance health and long life. As a result of these clinical and physiological findings, the minerals have been extensively promoted as "health-promoting" nutrients happen because of monetary reasons than their actual high worth of health and life-giving remedies mostly, by merchants, news media, and some health book authors (7, 8, 51, 52, 53, 55).

Also, nutrition experts and physicians have made many reports emphasizing on the beneficial impact on the use of minerals to prevent and effectively treat dreaded diseases namely, cancer, diabetes, heart diseases, cognitive function impairment or loss. There have been situations where some patients bring some of the minerals to Nutrition and Health Professional for simple clarification about them (7, 8, 51, 52, 53, 55).

Professional should seize an opportunity such as this as an avenue of health education and health promotion to enlighten the patients. Now that studies are discovering the efficacies or health benefits of the minerals, a discussion of the essentiality of functions of mineral to the body is now more necessary than ever (7, 8).

There are only five macro minerals or macro elements namely, potassium, sodium, calcium, magnesium, and phosphorus (KNaCaMgP). For body weight, calcium consist of 920 - 1200 g (1.5%) of human adult body weight. Human bone and teeth consist of 99% calcium (21). Phosphorus constitutes up to one percent of human body weight and 2/3 of calcium component of the body occur together with phosphorus. Although lots of trace elements abound in nutrition, only 10 are of specific biochemical functions namely, iron, iodine, copper, chlorine, sulphur, zinc, cobalt, selenium, molybdenum, and manganese (21).

There is a possibility that 15 trace elements are essentially needed in human body namely, lithium, lead, tin, flourine, chromium, vanadium, silicon, aluminum, arsenic, boron, bromine, germanium, cadmium, nickel, and rubidium. These 15 elements do not have a defined specific biochemical functions; however, there were studies that suggested that these elements are essential in certain circumstances (51, 52, 53, 55, 56).

Evidence suggesting nickel, silicon, chromium, boron, arsenic, and vanadium to be essential trace element are significant. Food and Nutrition Board stated that nutrients regarded as essential were established in 1940. Nutrients are chemical substances that are essential for life, growth and repair in the body (51, 52, 53, 55, 56). Those that the body can not manufacture they are regarded as essential-indispensable, a person has to consume them directly or substance from which the body can manufacture them - precursors (51, 52, 53, 55, 56).

When the body is deficient in any of those, it results in illnesses, or no, or low growth.

While some minerals, are required in comparatively low levels in the body, macrominerals are needed in larger quantities. The mineral needed in higher amount than others are called macrominerals and those required in minute quantities are named microminerals (51, 52, 53, 55, 56).

Food and Nutrition Board, described nutrients as chemical substances component of food essential for life, tissue growth and repair. The nutrients that the body cannot produce are called essential or indispensable nutrients because their deficiency in the body cause the body to develop diseases, prevent growth and in some cases cause death. Just like salt is fortified with iodine to address the problem of iodine deficiency and hypothyroidism, vitamin A, Zinc and Iron powder are now included in World Health Organization's essential medicines list to help address an issue of nutrients' deficiency among children in the developing countries (21, 51, 52, 53, 55, 56).

Attempts to Define the Word Essentiality

Following the animal growth model, essential nutrient was described in 1960-1970, deficiency of essential nutrients were described to prevent life cycle (growth, development, or maturation including reproduction) or cause death. Six conditions were indicated for an element to be regarded as essential among the condition is the sixth condition, which is that the element must cause a consistent adverse alteration of biological function from performing at optimal capacity, and such change could be prevented or reversed when the physiological quantity of the element is raised to normal or optimum (7, 8).

Currently, the most acceptable description of essential element is that it must have a definite biological function. As a result of the controversies between 1980s and 1990s over definition of essential element, there is no universally accepted list of essential elements (7, 8).

Terms used to Describe Nutritional Effects And Conditions of Essentiality

There are other terms used in nutrition to describe the effects of essential nutrients on human health. These are:

1. **Conditionally Essential Nutrient**: This means that a nutrient is generally not essential, which means that it is dispensable in some cases and indispensable in other cases. In certain pathological conditions, it is essential, or indispensable in some it is not essential. A conditionally essential nutrient must be presence in someone's diet for a maintenance of health for a specified demographics namely, certain age, specific stage of development, or certain

pathologic conditions (52, 53, 55). They perform specific essential type of function under certain environment, nutrition, hormone and physiology. Conditional essentiality usually involve organic compounds namely, glutamine and carnitine, usually synthesized in the body at low or optimum levels, and does not involve mineral elements (52, 53, 55).

2. **Pharmacological Effect**: This term is used to describe a fact that certain deficient nutrient has a capability to change biological structure, biochemical function when administered therapeutically. Common examples are seen in **lithium**, which has antimanic (preventing hyper, mania, madness, insanity) properties, and **fluoride**, which prevents demineralization of tissues caused by calcification or hardening.

3. **Nutritional Effect**: This term means that nutrient has an ability to restore deficient nutrient and restore nuriture when administered through diet but, not necessarily changing structure, biochemical and physiological function, as is true with pharmacological effect or benefit. Nutrient is beneficial when it can restore health after its intake is raised to optimum, and the restoration of health can consequently change the nutritional, physiological, hormonal, and metabolic stress, or impact (52, 53, 55). It is important to note that, if a nutrient is deficient or low, and there is no existing disease/s, or low essential nutrient intake that could impact negatively on someone, the body can cope with low level of nutrient, but presence of diseases, plus deficiency of other trace element could cause health problem (52, 53, 55).

4. **Nutritional Importance Beyond Essentiality**: Some nutrients may not be essential in diet but, they are nutritionally important. Certain nutrients not regarded as essential nutrients for example selenium, have been linked with promoting health and decreasing chronic diseases risks. Thus, the USA Food and nutrition Board came to a conclusion that it is necessary that a new concept targeted at reducing chronic diseases risk be included in future Recommended daily Allowance (RDA), and that concept is now called Dietary Reference Intake (DRI) (52, 53, 55). And this is taking nutrition to a new subject that is concerned with the total

health effect of nutrient to the body. Attention is required in the area of determining lower and upper limit for some RDA, and to make recommendation for elements or nutrients that are nutritionally essential or beneficial and are capable of reducing chronic disease risks, although, consistent evidence that support universally accepted definition of essentiality of nutrient is yet to be determined (52, 53, 55).

Thus, *directing attention on developing a universal definition of essential nutrient is a call to duty to all nutrition science professionals.* I hereby make an attempt to describe or define essentiality of nutrient. Based upon the knowledge gathered from this study this author therefore described an essential nutrient as: **A nutrient be it macro, micro or trace that when it is continuously missing in the body causes biological or biochemical, or physiological dysfunction, or causes the body tissues or structures to change conditions, which are preventable, had the nutrient been available at optimum level required to perform those functions, and it is a component of a necessary biological, and biochemical molecule at various stages and forms of life.**

Categorizing Possible Essential Trace Elements:

Evidence suggest that elements could possibly become essential if one or more of the following conditions are met:

1. When diet is deficient in trace element, it consistently cause biological function, body structure, or tissue composition to change, which is preventable, or reversible by mere intake of the deficient element to an optimum level.
2. It is required in specified concentration for a known biochemical function
3. It is part or component of a known importance biological molecule in some form of life.
4. It performs essential function in lower form of life (micro organisms).

Question 1
1. What does conditionally essentiality nutrient means?

Answer 1 It means that a nutrient is generally not essential in all conditions to all animals, but in certain pathological conditions, it is essential, or indispensable. A conditionally essential nutrient must be presence in someone's diet for a maintenance of health for a specified demographics namely, certain age, specific stage of development, or certain pathologic conditions. They perform specific essential type of function under certain environment, nutrition, hormone and physiology. Conditional essentiality usually involve organic compounds namely, glutamine and carnitine, usually synthesized in the body at low or optimum levels, and does not involve mineral elements.

Question 2
What is the most accepted definition of essential element?

Answer 2
An essential element must be cable of performing a definite biological function.

Question 3
What is the difference between Pharmacological effect and Nutritional effect

Answer 3 Pharmacological effect is a term used to describe a fact that certain deficient nutrient has a capability to change biological structure, biochemical function when administered therapeutically (by treatment). But for nutritional effect, it means that nutrient has an ability to restore deficient nutrient when administered through diet without necessarily changing structure, biochemical and physiological functions as seen in nutrient with pharmacological effect. Intake or eating of essential nutrient at optimum level can restore health in terms of changing the nutritional, physiological, hormonal, and metabolic stress, or impact

Minerals are inorganic substances that are essential to the body although, the body needs them regularly only in small quantities. It is necessary for the maintenance of acid-base balance in the body. That means minerals handle the controlling of alkaline (base), and acid condition of the body to keep it neutral. It is essential for the formation of blood cells, teeth and bone. Examples of essential minerals are phosphorus, calcium, sodium, magnesium, cobalt, chromium, iodine, fluoride, zinc, hydrochloric acid, molybdenum, selenium, potassium and iron, etc (52, 53, 55, 56, 57).

Keeping in mind the lesson of micronutrient mineral nuriture, and essentiality, below is a discussion about specific macrominerals, starting with sulfur.

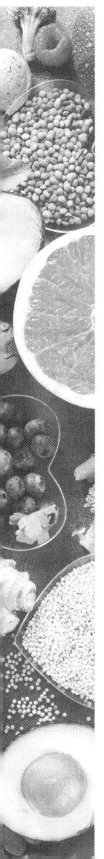

Chapter 13

Micromineral: Sulfur (S)

Sulfur is a key component of all proteins and it plays a major role in forming the body cells and in keeping the body safe from diseases, and toxic substances invasion. Sulfur is needed in the development and maintenance of the connective tissues and it is essential for the structural strength of the skin (51, 52, 53, 55).

Functions

Sulphur is a component of protein molecules that plays a key role in keeping the body safe from bacteria invasion as well as toxic substances. It is an essential element for healthy development of connective tissues, and to maintain the structural integrity of the skin.

Sources

Animal sources: meats: poultry, egg, fish, seafoods, oysters, lobsters, shrimps, and milk.

Plant Sources: Vegetables: leafy vegetables example fluted pumpkin leaves, bitter leaves, green tete, Kale, collard green, or red, egg-plant leaves, spinach, cruciferous plants example, cabbage, cauliflower, broccoli, Brussels sprouts, turnips, boo Choy, and kohlrabi. Others are allium crops namely, garlic, leek, onions, and chives. It is also present in nuts, and legumes (51, 52, 53, 55).

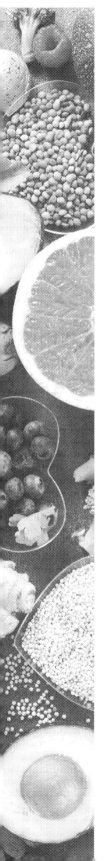

Chapter 14

Macrominerals: Magnesium (Mg)

Magnesium is a mineral element that is counted among the first 20 elements in the periodic table of chemistry. At birth, it occurs at a level of 760 mg, and it increases as one grows. Magnesium increases to 5g at age 4-5 months, and 25g at the age of 1-3 years. It is predominantly located in the skeleton accounting for 1% of bone ash, 30-40% in tissues and muscles, and 1% in extracellular fluids (52, 53, 55, 56, 59).

Function

As an enzyme cofactor, main function of magnesium in soft tissues is to support metabolic processes, manufacturing of proteins, RNA and DNA. It also supports the maintenance of electrical processes in the nerve tissues and cell membranes. When magnesium is low or deficient in the cells, potassium is also affected negatively, making it low too. Similar to potassium, when magnesium is low, calcium also goes low in the body (52, 53, 55, 56, 59, 60).

Magnesium is nicknamed "multipurpose mineral" It performs a broad range of functions in the body, and it facilitates over 300 biochemical reactions in the body, although, it is needed in minute (tiny) quantity. Quite like calcium, magnesium works jointly with Phosphorus, oxides, or nitrates before carrying out its numerous functions (52, 53, 55, 56, 60). It is a coenzyme factor that supports neurone chemical transmission, and muscular movements (59, 60).

Magnesium enhances nitric oxide production, inhibits reactive oxygen species (ROS), which are compounds containing harmful oxygen that are very reactive and unstable that cause cell oxidation and cell damage. Presence of antioxidants reverses and prevents cell oxidation caused by ROS examples of antioxidants are vitamins A, C and E and phytochemical compounds (50, 53, 55, 56, 60).

Recommendation

Up to 380 mg causes toxicity. 65 mg is good for children one to three years old, 110mg for children aged four to 10 and 350 mg for teenagers and adult. For Canadians, 20 mg per day is recommended Nutrition Intake (RNIs) for infants 0-4 months, 23 mg per day for infants aged five months to one year old, other countries' recommendation is higher than that of Canadian (51, 52, 53, 55, 59).

Functions

- Magnesium is an essential component of the bone.
- It is vital for protein synthesis, and contraction of the muscle and nervous transmission.
- It boosts the immune system, and aids in prevention of constipation.
- It promotes proper growth and maintains healthy bones.
- It is used as an antacid for indigestion caused by stomach acid.
- Enhances the central nervous system (CNS).
- It maintains healthy blood pressure and normal sugar level.
- It helps in the synthesis of protein.
- It enhances tolerance and endurance during sports and exercise.
- It improves mineral transportation in the blood
- It prevents the pile up of cholesterol in the tissues and hinders blockage of blood vessels with fat depositions and the possible heart attack.

Sign of Excess Magnesium Sulphate

- Alteration (changes) in electrocardiogram (ECG).
- Osteomalacia (bone demineralization), low mineral absorption of the bones, reduction in the density of the bone, or osteoporosis.
- Muscle weakness and hyperactivity.
- Obstruction of the intestine.
- It raises the heartbeats (51, 52, 53, 55).
- Excess magnesium sulphate causes hypotension or kidney disease.
- It causes the respiratory system to be stuffy and could cause chest pain.
- It has negative effects on the sight and it causes face flushing (increase in blood flow into the face as a result of heat or rise in temperature).
- It causes abnormal blood circulation (51, 52, 53, 55, 59).

Magnesium Deficiency

- Deficiency of magnesium alters the electrocardiogram (ECG).
- It lowers the density of the bone, and it causes osteoporosis.
- It causes muscle weakness and hyperactivity.
- It results in the obstruction of the intestine (51, 52, 53, 55, 59).
- It negatively affects the central nervous system (CNS).
- It reduces the heartbeat.
- It causes the respiratory system to be stuffy and could cause chest pain.
- It lowers the circulation of the blood and oxygen (51, 52, 53, 55, 59).

Food Sources

Magnesium is predominantly found in all green leafy vegetables such as fluted pumpkin leaves, spinach, bitter leave, green tete, okra and so forth. It could be found in legumes such as beans, and dairy products (milk products example ice cream and yogurt). Magnesium could be found in whole grains namely oat, and other sources such as cocoyam, fish, apricot, avocado pear, banana, raisins and peaches (51, 52, 53, 55, 59). All vegetables are better eaten uncooked or very slightly cooked with gentle heat with its green colour still intact. Taking the juice or extract of vegetables is nutritionally beneficial to health. Other sources of magnesium are lemon fruit, coconut juice, spices such as paprika, basil, peppermint, parsley, lemongrass. Others are Artichokes, walnuts, cashew nut, almonds, peanuts, pine, and Brazil nuts (51, 52, 53, 55, 59). Also, it is available in Kale, collard, cabbage, and Chinese broccoli. Remember Kale and collards green are among vegetable that require gentle cooking before eating. It could be obtained from drinking water, and chocolate bar.

Having learned about magnesium next, is about calcium.

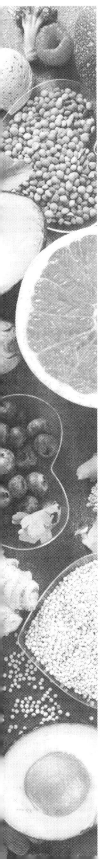

Chapter 15

Macromineral: Calcium (Ca)

Calcium never works alone, but rather works jointly with phosphorus as calcium phosphate in the presence of Vitamin D. Calcium occur abundantly in the body. It is mostly located in the bone and teeth, where it is naturally stored. It could be found in the muscle, blood, and in the intercellular fluids. Nearly 99% of calcium is stored in the teeth and bone (51, 52, 53, 55, 61, 62). Calcium level of uncultivated vegetables and fruits are as high as that of milk; hence, after weaning, infants are found to have calcium level higher than normal. There is low calcium in cereal grains that replaced uncultivated vegetables and fruits; however, consuming high amount of bioavailable milk calcium along side cereal grains makes up or complements for low calcium from cereal grains (51, 52, 53, 55).

Before old age or menopause, the formation of bone establishes a balance between calcium formation and calcium absorption. However, at old age, this balance faces some alteration, and often the calcium reabsorption and deposition rate changes. The breakdown of bone becomes higher than the rate at which it is formed (51, 52, 53, 55). The consequence is the loss of bone (osteoporosis). In early childhood the reverse is the case, the rate of bone formation is higher than the rate of its absorption. But, in the adolescent and people below menopause, the rate of bone formation is equal to the rate of its reabsorption. Meaning that absorption of 10 g of calcium in the later group will result in a formation of bone equivalent to 10 g (51, 52, 53, 55, 61, 62.).

Calcium Absorption and Bioavailability

Calcium absorption in the lumen of the intestine occurs through two major mechanisms and it is important in deterring the amount of calcium in the body namely, active trans-cellular absorption (TCA), which takes place in the duodenum when there is low level of calcium in the body, and passive paracellular absorption, occurring in the intestine/colon when there is moderate to high calcium in the body.

Active trans-cellular absorption (TCA) involves a number of processes. It starts by importing calcium into the enterocyte (intestine lining), from where it is transported across cells. Then, it is exported into the blood and extracellular fluids. Calcium can move within the epithelial cells of the intestine through voltage-insensitive channel. Calcium enzyme example ca2+, Na+, and K+- ATpase hydrolysis adenosinetriphosphate (ATP) to form adenosinediphosphate (ADP) to releases energy. To hydrolyze ATP the enzyme will simply remove one molecule of phosphorus from ATP and the enzyme is called adenosinetriphosphatase (ATPase). Also, ATPase pumps calcium, sodium and potassium ions in and out of the cells during metabolic processes in the mitochondria. Mitochondria is a place where large amount of energy is released to the body during the process of digestion. The same ATP enzyme (ATPase can also catabolize adenosinediphosphate and phosphate to form ATP. To catabolize simply means adding one molecule of phosphorus to ADP to form ATP (49, 50). Transportation of Calcium across epithelial cells places a limit to the level of active cellular absorption, and the presence of cal-binding (calcium binding) compound called D-dependant protein that binds calcium also, increases the limitations of active cellular calcium absorption in the body. Cal-binding protein cannot be produced without vitamin D.

Passive paracellular absorption (PCA): PCA occurs in the parts of the intestine called jejunum and ileum, and it can take place in the colon as well, when there is moderate to high level of calcium in the body moving through tight junctions to basolateral (polarized) regions of the enterocytes-lining of the intestine then, into the blood. Bulk absorption of Calcium occurs through PCA when Calcium level is high and a short time is needed for its absorption (51, 52, 53).

Functions

- Calcium is essential for a strong bone and teeth formation and bones.
- It is necessary for the relaxation and contraction of the muscles, and vital for nervous transmissions.
- Calcium plays an important role in boosting the immune system.
- And it is necessary for regulating the blood pressure and blood clotting (51, 52, 53, 55).
- It is also good for the nerves and the brain.
- Promotes the formation of calcium phosphate.
- Promotes the utilization of phosphorus in the body.
- Promotes the secretion of hormones.
- Promotes the function of the muscle.
- Promotes the exchange of signals between the cells.
- It is essential for the heart's vascular contraction, and vasodilation.
- It aids in keeping acid-alkaline balance in the body, thus maintaining the body PH (20, 61, 62).
- It promotes weight loss.
- It is essential for heart, muscle and digestive health
- It is required for strong bones.
- It is necessary for blood cells formation and synthesis

Deficiency

- Calcium deficiency causes loss of bone mass or osteoporosis.
- It lowers the formation of calcium phosphate
- It causes rickets formation or bone malformation Loss of bone mass or osteoporosis (20, 51, 52, 61, 62).
- It causes hypocalcaemia: blood calcium deficiency.

Toxicity

Excess consumption of calcium result in hypercalcaemia: Abnormal or excess calcium in blood circulation, it can cause kidney stone, weaken the bones and usually caused by overactive parathyroid gland. It also, interferes with the normal functions of the brain and heart (51, 52, 53, 55).

Food Sources

Animal Sources: Meat, poultry, cartilage, snail, mushroom, milk and dairy products such as cheese, and yoghurt.

Plant sources: are dark leafy green vegetables, such as fluted pumpkin leaves, Spinach, water leaves, green tete, kale, and collard. The food sources of calcium are spices such as basil, thyme, parsley and mint. Others are celery seeds, rosemary and quinoa. It could be found in fruits namely, orange and citrus as well as cabbage, and broccoli. Calcium is also obtainable from nuts namely, almonds, and beans, sesame seeds and chia seeds (61, 62).

With the lesson about calcium in thoughts next, is about phosphorus.

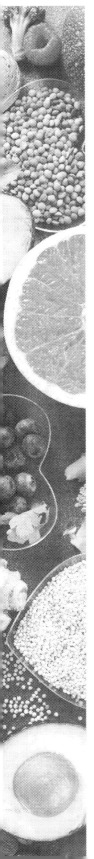

Chapter 16

Macromineral: Phosphorus (P)

It is vital for energy release and the utilization of carbohydrates, fats, vitamins and minerals in the body e.g. iron, magnesium, potassium, and sodium, etc. Just as mentioned above it performs best jointly with calcium as calcium phosphate. Good for strong and healthy teeth and bone. It controls the acid-base balance inside the body and the acidity (pH) of the blood, acting as a buffer. It facilitates the production of protein inside the body and promotes the growth and repair of worn out tissues (21, 60, 63, 64).

It improves the performance of Kidney and regulates the heartbeats. About 85% of the body phosphorus is present in the bone, and inside the body it is present as calcium phosphate. It is one of the components of Ribonucleic acid (RNA), and deoxyribonucleic acid (DNA). It is naturally attached to the red blood cell, and it promotes the circulation of oxygen to the body tissues (21, 60, 63, 64). In developing world where plants and vegetables constitute predominantly daily meal, the dietary phosphorus/calcium ratio is estimated at 1.6:1, and in colder regions of the world where animal products constitute daily meals, phosphorus/ calcium intake ratio is placed at about 4.5:1, which is greater than the former (developing world) (21, 60, 63, 64).

Functions

Phosphorus is found in all cells and it necessary for proper function of the all body cells. Just like zinc phosphorus is essential in many metabolic and developmental activities in the body. It is essential for protein synthesis, needed for growth, repair and maintenance of the body cells (21; 58.). It is a vital element for adenosine triphosphate (ATP), and energy production. Phosphorus helps to maintain healthy bones and teeth. It is necessary for the maintenance of acid-base balance in the body. Jointly with B group vitamins, phosphorus is essential for kidney functions, constriction of muscles, nervous transmission and regular heartbeat (21, 60, 63, 64).

- It regulates the amount of calcium in the body.
- It makes the bone, and the teeth strong (21, 60, 63, 64).
- It is essential during the metabolic process in the biochemical production of adenosine triphosphate (ATP). ATP is the body cell energy-giving molecule.
- It controls the acid-base balance inside the body and the acidity (PH) of the blood (58).
- It facilitates the production of the protein inside the body and promotes the growth and repair of worn out tissues.
- It improves the performance of kidney and regulates the heartbeats (60, 62, 64).

Deficiency of Phosphorus

Phosphorus is commonly present in many animal and plant foods. It is rare for the body to experience deficiency of phosphorus (21, 60, 63, 64); however, if the body lacks phosphorus it is called hypophosphatemia, and it causes poor appetite, anaemia, and poor immunity. It could manifest in rickets, which is a bone malformation. Deficiency of phosphorus also causes numbness, and muscle ache.

Toxicity

- Excessive intake of phosphorus is called hyperphosphatemia. It result in health risk, making the body to move calcium from bone to the blood to maintain a balanced phosphorus level in the body. The consequence of this action would be the weakness of the bone (21, 60, 63, 64).

Food Sources

Animal Sources: Fish, example salmon, tilapia, shellfish-scallops is an excellent source of phosphorus. It is also available in meat, poultry including egg, and milk and dairy products example, yogurt, ice cream, cheese.

Plant sources: are beans, nuts, cereals, and peas. Yeast is also a good source of phosphorus. Processed food such as soda, pop, and soy food example tofu are sources of phosphorus (21, 60, 63, 64).

Keeping in mind the lesson about phosphorus next, is about sodium.

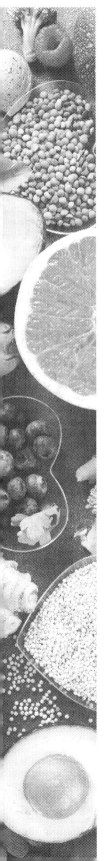

Chapter 17

Macromineral: Sodium (Na)

Function

It is essential for fluid and electrolyte balance in the body. It is important element for maintaining heart functions, specific metabolic functions, nerve transmission and muscle contraction (51, 52, 53, 55). Essential for ATP regulation, and electrolyte balance (21).

Deficiency

Results in hyponatremia: Sodium deficiency is rare because it is easily obtainable from table salt, Nacl, processed foods, animals and plants (21).

Toxicity

Manifested in hypernatremia: excess or abnormal blood sodium (21).

Sources

It is obtainable from table salt, bread, and abundance in processed foods namely, soy sauce, instant noodles, soups, or beef noodles, pastas, roasted and salted nuts, and seeds examples, peanuts, almonds, walnuts, cashew nuts, and pumpkin and melon seeds. It is high in fast foods such as ham, sausages, biscuits, and egg. Cured meats, fish, yogurt, milk, baked potatoes, and acorn squash. Fresh and dried fruits and vegetables, whole grans and legumes (51, 52, 53, 55, 59).

With the lesson about sodium in thoughts next, is about potassium.

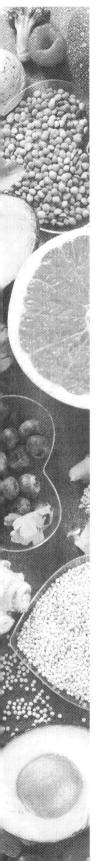

Chapter 18

Macromineral: Potassium (K)

Potassium is an essential macro mineral needed in the body in relatively large amount compared to micro minerals such as boron, copper and molybdenum

Function

Potassium is essential for maintaining the balance of fluid and electrolyte. It is necessary for healthy function of the heart, and specific metabolic functions. It is important for nerve transmission and contraction of the muscles. It is needed for the optimum maintenance of blood pressure and the removal of waste products from the body (51, 52, 53, 55, 59).

Sources

Animal sources: Meats, fish example, salmon, milk, and yogurt. It could be obtained from baked potatoes and acorn squash. **Plant**: Vegetables and fruits: Fresh and dried vegetables and fruits, whole grains, and legumes examples beans, lentils, and peas (51, 52, 53, 55, 59).

Having learned about potassium next, is about microminerals, starting with aluminium.

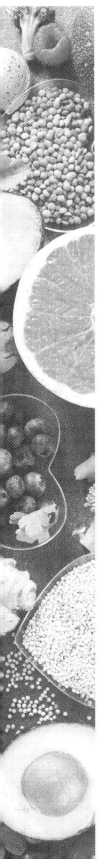

Chapter 19

Microminerals: Aluminum (Al)

Deficiency of aluminum in goat cause increase in abortion, hind legs weakness, incoordination and low life expectancy, depression of growth in chicken. It activates fluoride of guanine nucleotide-binding regulation of adenylate cyclase-an enzyme that plays a regulatory or control function in the body cell (52, 53, 55, 56, 59).

When aluminium toxicity is severe such as seen in dementia, and in dialysis, it could manifest in seizure, disorientation, hallucination, and speech disturbances. Aluminum toxicity can cause toxicity of the neurone, and adverse change in the skeleton. Toxicity of the skeleton cause pain in bone and bone fracture (52, 53, 55, 56, 59).

Functions

Aluminium activates fluoride of guanine nucleotide-binding protein (G proteins) regulation of adenylate cyclase. G protein switches molecules inside the cells. G-proteins receives signals from interior cells and sends it to exterior cells and vice versa (52, 53, 55, 56, 59).

It stimulates the production of DNA, and the activation of G-protein to prompt bone formation of osteoblasts (bone structure formation). It helps to prevent Alzheimers and dementia diseases.

Deficiency

Deficiency will result in low blood aluminium level, which can hamper its functions as mentioned above (52, 53, 55, 56).

Toxicity

When toxicity is severe such as seen in dementia, in dialysis, it could manifest in seizure, disorientation, hallucination, and speech disturbances. Alzheimer's disease was linked to aluminum toxicity. Kidney dialysis, and tubal feeding could cause aluminum toxicity It can result in the toxicity of the skeleton causing pain in bone and bone fracture (52, 53, 55, 56, 59).

Food Sources

Baked food produced with chemical raising agents such as baking powder, processed cheese, herbs, tea, grains, and vegetables.

Keeping the lesson about aluminium in thoughts next, is about Arsenic.

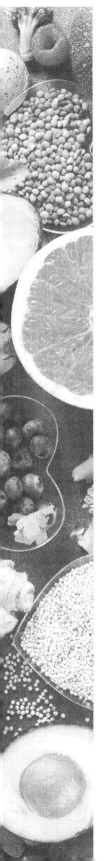

Chapter 20

Micromineral: Arsenic (As)

Arsenic performs an essential role in human because individuals with cancer, central nervous system, and vascular injuries manifested low blood arsenic level. Deficiency of arsenic alters the ratio of S-adenosylmethionine/S-adenosylhomocysteine of the body tissue to low and a reduction in the ratio was linked to DNA hypomethylation (low ability to add methyl group to DNA) that causes some kind of cancer in humans. S-adenosylmethionine/S-adenosylhomocysteine inhibits or prevents enzyme functions in the DNA that are responsible for methylation in the DNA. An example of the enzyme is methyltransferase. Methylation is a process of replacing hydrogen in the DNA with alkyl groups or atom example, methyl. Arsenic is an essential trace element to humans (52, 53, 55, 56, 59). Arsenic can be substituted in place of phosphate to activate certain enzymes or metabolites. It induces some kind of protein responsible for stress or heat shock. It increases methylation-methy formation, and DNA production in human lungs and lymphocytes (52, 53, 55, 56).

Recommended Dietary Allowance (RDA)

Recommended intake is 0.3 microgram (ug)/kg body weight, or 21 microgram (ug) per 70 kg body weight of a person.

Upper limit is 140-250 microgram (ug) per day. Average recommended intake from across the globe is 12-60 microgram (ug) per day. For united states, 30 microgram (ug) per day is recommended (52, 53, 55, 56).

Deficiency

Deficiency cause low growth, abnormal reproduction, fertility problem, parental- death of young shortly before birth or after birth in rat, goat and pig. Deficiency in goat specifically result in low triglycerides, myocardial infarction-heart attack (sudden cutting off of blood flow to the heart muscle and causing tissue damage) and death of lactating mother goat. It can cause high mineral level of organs and calcification of kidney. It can cause methylation that can cause high level of arsenic in the urine (52, 53, 55, 56).

Upper Limits (ULs) intake: maximum acceptable intake of certain essential micronutrients from water, food, and supplement that may not cause toxicity or adverse health effect on the body. Healthy range of micronutrients stays within the range of recommended nutrient intakes (RNIs) and the ULs, to be sufficient to protect the body from diseases, and to prevent toxicity.

Keeping the lesson of Arsenic in mind, next, is about boron.

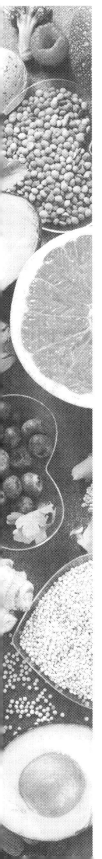

Chapter 21

Micromineral: Boron (B)

Essentiality of boron for lower animals is selective but for higher animals it is established because boron is required for a completion of fish life cycle. **A natural boron in bacteria produce antibiotics** and that in plant wall produce an organic complex compound called bis (rhamnogalacturonan-II) borate (52, 53, 55, 56).

Boron is involved in a number of enzymic activities in vitro animals, prompting a hypothesis that boron regulates metabolic reaction made possible by its component of hydroxyl containing reactant called substrate. Deficiency of boron has been linked to the impairment of calcium and energy metabolism, as well as the function of the human brain (52, 53, 55, 56).

Boron is linked with cadmium distribution regulation in the body.

Functions

It controls the effect of magnesium and phosphorus to improve estrogen level in post menopause women, which promotes healthy bones, and brain function. It aids the elimination of yeast infection in the vagina, and promotes healthy development of the embryo. It aids cells and organ membrane activities. It promotes the distribution of cadmium in the body 51, 52, 53, 55).

Sources

Plant Sources: Fruits and vegetables: examples, carrot, onions, broccoli, bananas, potatoes, peaches, pears, red grapes, apple, avocado, olives, dried fruits, namely, prunes, and rosins. It is also found in nuts especially almonds, coconuts, hazelnuts, walnuts, peanuts, legumes such as, beans, and lentils. Wheat, and oat bran. Other sources are, bee pollen, fruit juices and honey (51, 52, 53, 55).

With the lesson about boron, next, is about cadmium.

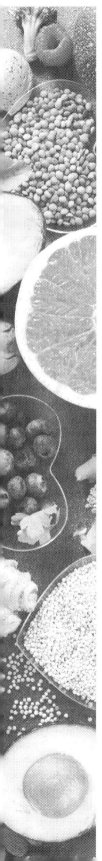

Chapter 22

Micromineral: Cadmium (Cd)

Cadmium has a long half-life in human body, and it causes depletion of essential minerals namely, zinc, calcium, copper, and iron in the body. It has high toxicity and only low quantity is needed and it could easily accumulate to prompt damage to organs, and renal dysfunction. It is toxic to kidney. Overdoes of cadmium can be toxic causing high blood pressure, osteomalacia-bone softening and deficiency of calcium or vitamin D, and some kind of cancer. World Health organization upper limit for cadmium is 70 microgram (ug) per day for a person who has 70kg body weight. Averagely, 10-20 microgram (ug) per day is a typical daily intake (52, 53, 55, 56)

Sources

Grains grown in cadmium rich soil, shellfish and vegetable leaves.

Next is about chloride.

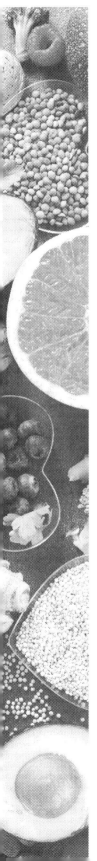

Chapter 23

Micromineral: Chloride (Cl)

Often occur together with sodium as sodium chloride, consisting of 40% sodium and 60% Chloride (table salt). It can be obtained from evaporated ocean or sea water. Depending on the source of salt, sometimes it can consist of traces of some minerals as zinc, iron and potassium (51, 52, 53, 55). For example Parkistani Himalaya salt in addition to sodium and chloride, consist of iron, potassium, calcium, and magnesium. It is pink in colour because it contains some oxides of iron as well. Also, chloride can occur as zinc chloride or hydrogen chloride (51, 52, 53, 55).

Functions

Chloride is an essential element necessary for the maintenance of fluid balance. Chloride is critically needed in the stomach juice for food digestion. It is essential for the production of hydrochloric acid needed for digestion essentially, protein, and fat digestion (21).

Deficiency

Deficiency of Chloride results in hypochloremia: low level or deficiency of chlorine in the blood.

Toxicity

Abnormal or high level of chlorine in the blood (21).

Sources

Animal sources: meats, and small quantity from milk.

Plant sources: celery, lettuce, seaweed, rye, tomatoes, and olives. Table salt (Nacl) is main source of chlorine and sodium. Processed foods contain large amount of chloride example bread, pasta, sausages, list is endless.

Having learned about chloride, next is about cobalt.

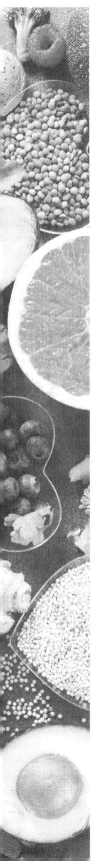

Chapter 24

Micromineral: Cobalt (Co)

Cobalt is a component of vitamin B12. Cobalt is essential for the formation of red blood cells and for anemia prevention. It is essential for inhibition of digestion, neurone, and muscle diseases (51, 52, 53, 55).

Functions

It is an essential component of vitamin B12 thus, it is necessary for the prevention of pernicious anemia. It promotes increases in blood level and formation of red blood cells (erythrocyte). Cobalt prevents fatigue, neuromuscular issues and digestive problem (51, 52, 53, 55).

Toxicity

Results in blood cobalt poisoning

Sources

Plant Sources: Fruits and Vegetables examples, cereals-oat, and millet; nuts example cashew nuts, peanuts, almonds, walnuts, and coconuts. Found in vegetables examples, mushrooms, green pepper, apple, bananas, broccoli, lettuce, and cabbage.

Animal sources: meat, kidney, liver, seafoods example oysters, lobsters, shrimps, mussels, fish and shellfish. Milk is also a good source of cobalt (51, 52, 53, 55). Keeping the lesson of cobalt in mind, next is about copper. Keeping the lesson of cobalt in mind, next, is about copper.

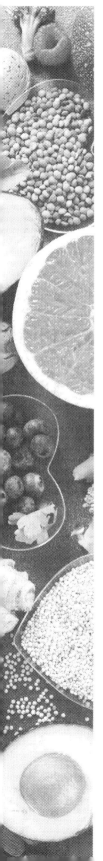

Chapter 25

Micromineral: Copper (Cu)

Copper is a component of many enzymes and it is composed of many enzyme structure. It is an essential trace elements. It is essential for metabolic processes and organ activities. It is a powerful immune booster. Copper neutralizes free radicals and prevents the body from oxidative stress damage (51, 52, 53, 55).

Functions

Copper is essential in the formation and maintenance of many enzyme structures. It is necessary for the metabolism of protein and iron. It promotes the function of many organs, and body metabolic processes. It boosts the immune system to prevent infectious diseases invasion into the body (51, 52, 53, 55). Just like zinc, copper **promotes the healing of wound and repair of injured tissues**. It prevents activities of free radicals by neutralizing it thus, preventing the body from the damage of oxidative stress. It is involved in redox enzyme reactions such as cytochrome C oxidase (51, 52, 53, 55).

Deficiency

Low blood copper

Toxicity

High or abnormal blood copper

Sources

Plants: Fruits and vegetables: cooked legumes example beans and chickpeas, nuts example cashew nuts, seeds example melon, sesame, and whole grains. Fluted pumpkin leaves, green tete, gongronema latifolium, bitter leaves, egg-plant leaves, raw kale, collards green, cooked mushrooms, avocado, and fermented soya beans food.

Animal Sources: organ meat, cooked seafoods, examples, oysters, shrimps, and lobster. Copper is also present in drinking water (51, 52, 53, 55).

Next is about chromium.

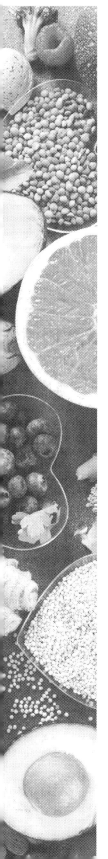

Chapter 26

Micromineral: Chromium (Cr)

Chromium is an essential trace element with a defined biochemical activities. There is a significant evidence suggesting nickel, silicon, chromium, boron, arsenic, and vanadium to be essential trace element are significant (52, 53, 55, 56). Chromium is essential in carbohydrate and fatty acids metabolism, synthesis of cholesterol and fatty acids and sugar regulation.

Functions

It is essential in the metabolism of carbohydrates and fats. It is necessary for brain functions, and body metabolic processes. It initiates the synthesis of cholesterol and fatty acids. It takes part in sugar regulation in the body together with the insulin (51, 52, 53, 55).

Deficiency

Low blood chromium

Toxicity

High blood chromium, which is harmful to the body.

Sources

Animals Sources: egg, beef, liver, poultry, oysters, cheese, butter, and unrefined or processed foods.

Plant sources: Fruits and Vegetables: black pepper, molasses, spinach, bananas, apple, green peppers, wheat germ, whole grains and nuts (51, 52, 53, 55).

With the lesson of chromium in mind, next, is about fluorine.

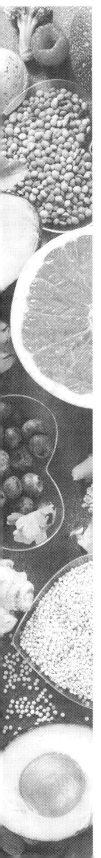

Chapter 27

Micromineral: Fluorine (F)

Evidence of essentiality of fluorine as a trace element is circumstantial. Deficiency of fluorine cause low growth rate in rat, and reduce life expectancy in goat. Flourine deficiency cause kidney and endocrine organs diseases. When rats and mice that have deficiency of iron were administered with fluorine, they experienced increase in blood cell production, growth, and fertility (52, 53, 55, 56).

It also inhibited teeth and bone demineralization, and nephrocalcinosis- high calcium deposition in kidney caused by high phosphorus. Fluorine occurs predominantly (99%) in tissue minerals as fluoroappetite, and it activates activities of some enzymes namely, adenylate cyclase (52, 53, 55, 56).

High dose of fluorine prevents dental caries. A suggestion that high fluorine intake could increase bone density and prevent osteoporosis is yet under investigation; so far, evidence is limited. In Tanzania, south Africa, China and India, it was reported that chronic high accumulation of fluorine is causing osteomalacia, osteoporosis, and osteosclerosis. Fluorine is not an essential trace element but, it has pharmacological value ((52, 53, 55, 56).

Adequate intake of fluorine for adult male is, 3.1 mg per day and adult female is 3.8 mg daily. Upper Limit intake for adult is 10mg daily.

Functions

Essential for the development of teeth and bone, prevents tooth decay, reduces cavities in children by half if their drinking water is treated with fluoride. Fluoride is essential in maintaining bone structure and slows the rate at which bone density is lost.

Sources

Fluorine occurs naturally in **Plants** example, it occurs in various types of tea, and in animal products.

Animal sources: seafoods example shellfish, and fish, deboned meat and poultry. Drinking water, and it is commonly found in foods. About 52% of united States fluorine come from water containing 0.7-1 2 mg per litre. Foodstuff sold in USA consist of 0.3-0.6 mg of fluoride daily intake.

Keeping the lesson about fluorine in thoughts next is about germanium.

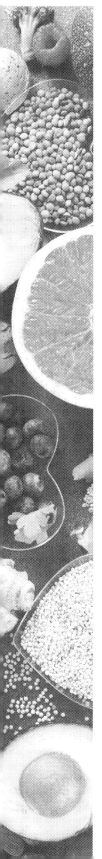

Chapter 28

Micromineral: Germanium (Gm)

In rat, there were circumstances where rat shin bone DNA was reduced owing to germanium deficiency, and germanium deficiency caused change in liver and bone minerals of the rat. Germanium intake also, reversed changes suffered as a result of deficiency of silicon, and some organic compound of germanium manifested ability to **prevent tumour** (anti-tumour) (52, 53, 55, 56).

High combustion of inorganic compound of germanium is toxic and can cause kidney damage. There are untested claims that organic germanium compounds namely, carboxyl ethyl germanium sesquioxide (Ge-132), and lactate-citrate germanate marked as nutritional supplement have immune boosting and anticancer properties (52, 53, 55, 56).

Dietary intake of germanium ranges from 0.4-1.5 mg per day per a person.

Sources

Wheat bran, vegetables, legumes and vegetables are rich sources of germanium.

Having learned about germanium next is about iodine.

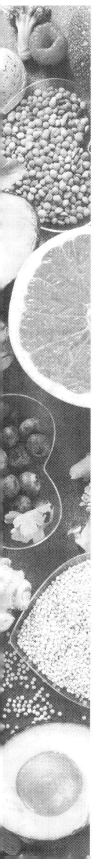

Chapter 29

Micromineral: Iodine (I)

Iodine is counted among the trace elements critical and major metabolic and cell processes in the human body. It is located largely in the thyroid, and blood. Iodine is needed in the human body for development, growth, metabolism, reproduction, muscle and nervous system functions.

Functions

Iodine is found in the thyroid hormone that thyroid gland makes and it plays a central role in major activities that take place in the human body namely, development, growth, metabolism, and reproduction. It is essential in the activities of the muscle and nerves, manufacture of blood cells, and the rate or speed of body metabolic processes. It is also involved in body temperature regulations (21, 51, 52, 53, 55).

Deficiency

Causes hypothyroidism, low blood iodine and it hinders all the metabolic processes and body functions indicated the function of iodine (21).

Toxicity

Causes hyperthyroidism or overactive parathyroid, which can cause kidney stone, weakness of the bones, and interfere with the normal activities of the brain and the heart (21).

Food Sources

Plant Sources: Fruits and Vegetables: All plants grown in a land rich in Iodine namely, bananas, cranberries, organic-grown naturally in the soil under sun and natural environments, organic strawberries, navy beans, and potatoes, dry prunes, *Chrysophillum Albidum (uda), cashew nut and leaves*. Others are African walnut, beet roots, kale, collard green

Animal sources: Seafoods namely, cod fish, lobster, and shrimps. **Dairy and milk products**: milk, organic cheese, cheddar cheese, baked turkey breast, and boiled egg. Others are iodized salt, and bread, canned tuna and corn, and baked potatoes (51, 52, 53, 55).

With the lesson of iodine in mind, next is about iron.

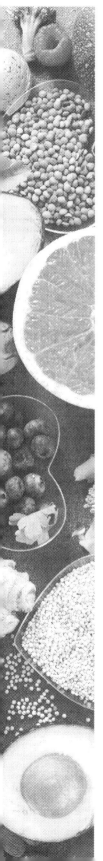

Chapter 30

Micromineral: Iron (Fe)

Iron is an essential trace element, and component of the blood, occurring widely and naturally in all animal products, dark-green leafy vegetables, nuts, legumes and fruits and seeds. It forms part of many enzymes like zinc, and other elements occurring as component of enzymes. It is a primary component of blood and enzymes. It is essential for synthesis of hemoglobin (51, 52, 53, 55).

Bioavailability and Absorption

Absorption of adequate amount of iron in the duodenum is essential. This high requirement of iron absorption from diet in the duodenum is negatively affected by presence of substances that interfere with the secretion of gastric acids example antacids (51, 52, 53, 55). Also, presence of chelating agent inhibits the absorption of iron. For a reason that women loss large quantity of iron during menstrual period, women have four times more iron transporters than men. Through active transport and under acidic conditions, iron is absorbed in the mucosal cells for the production of hemoglobin. For iron storage, a type of protein called ferritin protein bonds with ion of iron (fe^{2+} fe^{+3+}) (51, 52, 53, 55).

This function is made possible by ferrous enzyme located in the lumen of duodenum called ferrireductase reducing fe^{3+} to fe^{2+}. A divalent metal transporter together with ferritin protein is co-transported into the enterocytes. Divalent metal transporter transports not only iron but also, other divalent metals (51, 52, 53, 55). There are two pathways or processes involved in iron distribution inside the enterocytes. These pathways are affected by the complexity of the cell programming consisting of levels of iron in the diet and in the system, they are:

I. When there is abundance of iron in the enterocytes, it is held up (trapped) by ferritin protein, which makes it unavailable for absorption because it could not be transported into the blood. So, it is lost whenever the enterocytes die.

II. This occurs when there is low level of iron in the body by an iron protein transporter in the basolateral membrane, where it is transported all through the body by iron carrier called transferrin (51, 52, 53, 55). Also, Iron can get into the body in the form of heme-fe from digested hemoglobin and myoglobin in the enterocytes of the small intestine made possible by an active transporter called endocyose. Once inside the enterocytes, Iron is freely available for absorption including inorganic iron (51, 52, 53, 55).

Hepcidin is a tiny peptide that regulates iron in the body, and this tiny peptide consists of 25 amino acids that regulates the homeostasis-iron: fluid balance in the body. Cytokines specifically interleukin(IL)-6, which inhibits inflammation regulates the releases of hepcidin (51, 52, 53, 55). Also involved in the regulation or adjustment of release of hepcidin are amount of iron required in the formation of erythrocytes (red blood cells), and level of iron in iron-reservoirs, as well as liposaacharide of bacteria. When hepcidin interacts with transmembrane portion called ferroportin it makes ferroportin in membrane of enterocyte, macrophage, and hepatocyte inactive, hence, causing low iron metabolism. Through iron storage, absorption, and recycling, excess iron can be brought to normal (51, 52, 53, 55).

Inflammation, and infectious diseases can lower iron absorption because it raises hepcidin level, when responding to acute-phase reaction caused by inflammation. This high amount of hepcidin brakes down the ferroportin causing the regulatory iron hormones to clog the path from, which iron is moved from the wall of intestine to the blood plasma (51, 52, 53, 55). The result of this action is increase in the immune system, and blocking of diseases pathogens, and infectious diseases growth, through curtailing of the supply of iron to plasma.

Lowering hepcidin production rate can be achieved by enhancing iron absorption of enterocytes, macrophages iron re-cycling, and iron storage in the hepatocyte, and it causes high level of iron release and absorption (51, 52, 53, 55).

Functions

Iron is a central element in the formation of hemoglobin (blood) in the human body cells. Iron transports oxygen from the lungs to the heart and from the heart to all around the body cells. As it is a component of the blood, and enzymes (49). It is essential for energy generation in the metabolic processes. It is involved in the distribution of electrons and electrolytes around the body cells. Like zinc, molybdenum and selenium it is a component of many enzymes, thus it is involved in enzyme functions in the body (51, 52, 53, 55).

Deficiency

Often iron deficiency results from its insufficient absorption and it causes anemia.

Toxicity

Excess iron in the body can be toxic to the body, reason is that mammals have no pathway for removal of excess iron. It cause an overload or access of iron in the blood (21).

Food Sources

Fruits and Vegetables:
    Plant sources: dark green leafy vegetables example: fluted pumpkin

leaves, kale, spinach, collards green and red, Swiss chard, green tete, egg-plant leaves, fruit, and cucumber; beans example, lima, brown, and black-eyed beans, lentils, peas, and white beans. Nuts and pulses- cashew, pine, hazel, peanut, almonds, pecan, walnuts. Others are dark chocolate, chocolate powder, and iron-enriched bread, tofu, and cereals.

Animal sources: animal products namely, chicken, turkey, lamb, goat, beef, liver, egg, milk, fish, mussels, bass. It is commonly found in foods; particularly plant foods (49).

Keeping the lesson of iron in thoughts next, is about lead

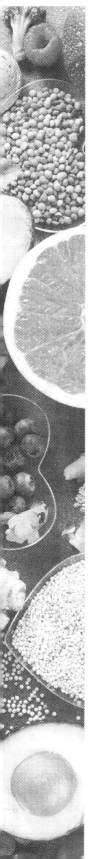

Chapter 31

Micromineral: Lead (Ld)

There were some evidence that supported that deficiency of lead caused changes in animal model used for experiment, and many evidence suggested that lead deficiency caused low growth and anemia, high blood cholesterol, phospholipids, and bile acids in rat. Deficiency of lead also interfered with iron metabolism, lowered the concentration of glucose, triglycerides, low density lipoprotein (LDL), and phospholipid in the liver (52, 53, 55, 56).

Additionally, researchers suggested that low lead result in rise in liver cholesterol, change in liver and blood enzymes. Consuming lead supplement was supported by evidence that it improved suboptimal growth in rat and alleviated deficiency of iron. Lead is involved in many biochemical activities in vitro. It is an essential biological element for lower form of life (52, 53, 55, 56).

Owing to toxicity and pollution linked with lead and the environment, attention given to lead is directed at it as pollutant and toxic element. Examples, are lead in paint and fuel additives. Least attention is given to lead as an element with nutritional value (52, 53, 55, 56).

Toxicity

Toxicity of lead cause, anemia, kidney damage, central nervous system abnormalities namely, subtle intelligence quotient (IQ), ataxia (abnormal and uncoordinated movements), convulsion and coma. High consumption of lead cause impaired motor function and lowers intelligence in children. **Deficiency of iron and calcium make toxicity of lead worse.** Lead is essential; however, toxicity is of huge concern. Estimated reference safe intake of lead is 5-50 microgram (ug) per day per person (52, 53, 55, 56).

Food Sources

Sea foods and plant food grown on soil rich in lead are rich food sources of lead.

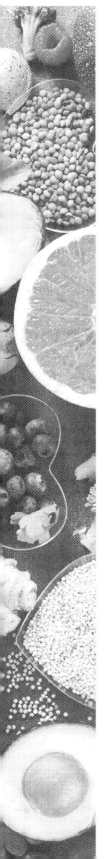

Chapter 32

Micromineral: Lithium (Li)

Lithium is not a categorized micromineral trace element, but it has pharmacological value, and it has profound anti-manic (mental health benefit preventing madness). Evidence suggested that people who drank water with low lithium level manifested high rate of violence crime. Lithium is not essential to lower form of animals, but it is essential for some biological processes of some form of life such as human beings (52, 53, 55, 56).

Recommended intake is 200 - 600 microgram (ug) per day per person.

ug: Microgram

Function

Lithium is involved in several blood, and liver enzyme activities. Rat fed with low lithium diet manifested low aggression and delayed amplitude of wheel-running (too much running around). Lithium is important for some cultured cells and has an ability to mimic insulin properties to prevent diabetes. It is essential for good physical, and mental health in mammals (21, 56).

Deficiency

Deficiency of lithium cause low fertility and birth weight in rat, as well as low weaning weight of young and litter size. It can cause poor mental health function in mammals (21, 56).

Toxicity

It is worthy of note that the margin between lithium doses and toxicity is too narrow hence, a major danger about using it to treat mental illness or madness. Mild lithium toxicity can result in, muscle weakness, tremor, feeling of dazed, drowsiness, gastrointestinal disorders, and severe toxicity can result in convulsion, coma, and death (19, 56).

Food Sources

Egg, fish, milk, and milk products, vegetables, potatoes, and processed meat. Remember that a significant amount of processed food including processed meat are not healthy food.

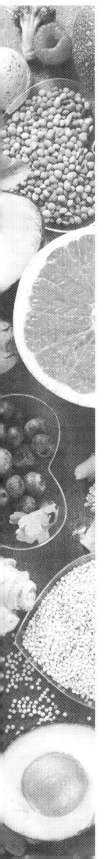

Chapter 33

Micromineral: Manganese (Mn)

Manganese is an essential trace mineral. It performs a general function as an enzyme co-factor and it is also a component of many enzymes. It is necessary for bone health and bone function (21, 19).

Functions

Promotes normal functioning of the human brain, and nervous system. Like zinc and molybdenum. Manganese is a component of many enzymes. Manganese is essential in the growth of bone, structure, and health. Manganese performs beneficial function to women that has past menopause, and prevents osteoporosis (51, 19).

Deficiency

Hypomagnesmia: Low magnesium in the blood, which will affect its functions mentioned above (21).

Toxicity

Hypermagnesemia: Abnormal or high blood magnesium is harmful to the body (21).

Food Sources

Plant Sources: Fruits and Vegetables: Cooked leafy vegetables example: fluted pumpkin leaves, kale, spinach, collards green and red, Swiss chard, green tete, egg-plant leaves, and cucumber; cooked beans example, lima beans, brown and black-eyed beans, fluted pumpkin seed, whole-grains example, brown rice, whole-wheat bread, tofu, and brewed black tea.

Animal sources: animal products namely, cooked fish, mussels, bass. It is commonly found in foods; particularly plant foods (51, 19).

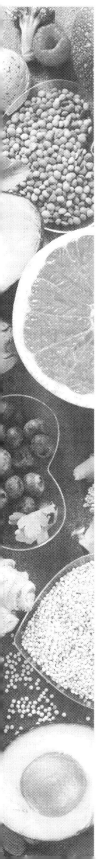

Chapter 34

Micromineral: Molybdenum (Mo)

It is one of the essential elements that has high value. The absorption and concentration of molybdenum is affected by calcium level in the body. It is counted among chelating metals. Molybdenum is a component of an enzyme called Xanthine oxidase (19, 54). Molybdenum is a component of many enzymes, and it is involved in many metabolic activities and enzyme functions (51; 19).

Functions

As a component of enzymes, it plays a central role in cell production through the activities of blood enzymes, and in the production and expending of energy in the mitochondria, which is the central energy source or powerhouse of the cells jointly with digested micronutrients. Molybdenum is also essential for the enzyme needed for the removal of waste products from the body (19, 51).

Deficiency

Low blood molybdenum, which could hamper its functions as mentioned above.

Toxicity

High, excess or abnormal blood molybdenum, and it can be harmful to the body.

Sources

Plant Sources: Fruits and vegetables, legumes-beans, lentil, and peas. From whole-grains, chokeberry, and leafy vegetables, Swiss chard, cucumber, sunflower seeds, wheat flour. **Animal sources**: liver, milk, cheese, organ meat, egg, and milk. Others are, bread, pasta-spaghetti, and macaroni (19, 51).

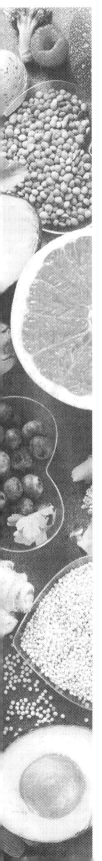

Chapter 35

Micromineral: Nickel (Ni)

Essentiality of nickel is significance but, circumstantial in animal species namely, goat chicken, cow, pig, sheep, and rat. Low growth, reproduction and blood sugar was manifested in rat and goat with nickel deficiency. Deficiency of nickel effects iron, calcium and zinc distribution in vitro. Effects of low nickel is mediated by presence of low or optimum levels of folic acid and vitamin B12 (19, 56). In anaerobic microorganisms, nickel is needed for hydrogenation, carboxylation, and desulfurization of enzymes. Nickel is located in the blood macroglobulin called nickeloplasmin.

Nickel initiates activities of many enzymes and promote the functions of folic acid and B12, and high level of vitamins B9 (folic acid) and B12 increase cardiovascular disease risk, and high dose of folic acid lowers the risk of neural tube defect in the new born (19, 56). Nickel performs a function of maintaining acid-base balance in human body. A relatively low intake of Nickel can affect the body adversely. Estimated safe daily intake of nickel obtained from animal experiment Model is 25 - 35 microgram (ug) per person per day, Upper limit of intake is tentatively suggested as below 600 microgram (ug) per person per day (19, 56).

Food Sources

Nuts, dry beans, chocolate, grains, and peas.

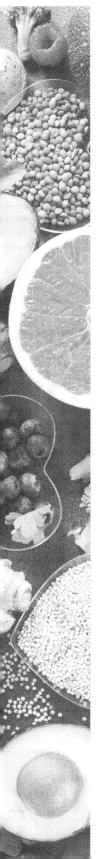

Chapter 36

Micromineral: Rubidium (Rb)

There is limited evidence supporting that rubidium is essential in certain circumstances. In goat, rubidium deficiency was reported to cause low food intake (appetite for food), growth, and life span. Also, it caused more cases of spontaneous abortion among pregnant goats. Rubidium could be used to replace potassium in some specified activities in the body of lower animals (19, 56). Rubidium has been linked to certain physiological activities of some neurones example, it is involved in the replacement of norepinephrine and electrical activities called electroencephalogram in the brain. Rubidium is not essential to lower forms of life, and it is not toxic. It is not an essential trace element but, it has beneficial effects to some lower form of animals thus, it has a potential to be beneficial to higher animals (19, 56).

About 1-5mg per person per day is considered safe, and adequate.

Food sources

Vegetables including asparagus, poultry, coffee, and black tea.

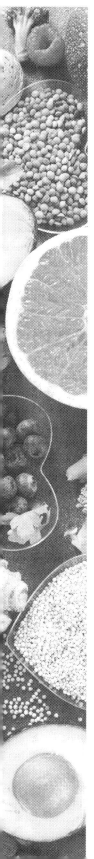

Chapter 37

Micromineral: Selenium (Se)

Selenium is an essential trace element for humans, rats and farm animals. Certain diseases have been implicated on the account of selenium deficiency. It protects the human body from oxidative-stress; stress occurring due to cell oxidation, offers protection to the body against diseases infection, and modulating growth and biological development. (52, 53, 55, 56). Selenium occurs predominantly in proteins in the form of selenoanalogues of amino acids, sulphides as selenotrisulphides. It could occur as acid-labile compound of selenium. About 30% of tissue selenium is coated in the muscle, liver containing 15%, and blood plasma containing 10%.

There are about 15 selenoproteins, with a concentration of 60-80% in blood plasma. It occurs as component of enzymes namely, glutathione peroxidase, and thioredoxin reductase, and these perform a function of balancing very reactive metabolites (enzymes) that contain oxygen. It protects the cells against infections by boosting cell immunity. Selenium enzyme called Glutathione peroxidase (GSHPx) helps with stress, infection, injury of the tissue, and protects the body tissues against harmful effect of oxygen-rich free radicals and hydrogen peroxide causing the destruction of the free radicals and the peroxides (52, 53, 55, 56).

Deficiency

Deficiency of selenium results in low blood glutathione peroxidase in mothers breast feeding for a long period of time (10 months and above). Infant formulae for babies five to eight months old and older was found to be low in selenium and that caused low selenium on the babies and that prompted recommendation of fortification of infant formulae with 10 microgram (ug) per day (52, 53, 55, 56). Less than 10 microgram (ug) of selenium in infants was implicated in cause of congestive heart failure, muscle weakness and myalgia- muscle pain, and when placed on selenium, recovered rapidly.

Keshan disease of Chinese children aged two to 10 years causing them fatigue after mild exercise, loss of appetite, cardiac arrhythmia (irregular or abnormal heart beat), cardiac insufficiency, cardiomegaly (enlarged heart or heart failure), and congestive heart failure were linked with selenium deficiency (52, 53, 55, 56). It resulted in multifocal myocardial necrosis (heart organ tissue death) and fibrosis, without affecting the coronary arteries. If selenium deficiency is detected early- three months earlier prior to myocardial infarction, administration of selenium can reverse the situation but, once, the diseases is established administration of selenium makes no difference (52, 53, 55, 56).

Adult estimated requirement of selenium is 7.4 -80 microgram (ug) per day. Upper limit of daily requirement for adult is 400 microgram (ug) per day, animals 2mg per kilogram dry diet for domesticated animals. No upper limited yet for children, pregnant, and lactating mothers. environment and agricultural practices affects food content of selenium (52, 53, 55, 56).

Absorption and Bioavailability

Absorption of selenium is not controlled by balance control, and it is readily absorbed by humans. Selenium of Brazilian nuts and kidney of beef is easily available and absorbed up to 90%, followed that of wheat 80%, sea foods namely, shrimp, herring, and crab; then, tuna which is is 20-60% (52, 53, 55, 56).

Function

It produces special proteins called antioxidants enzymes to protect the body against negative effect of heavy metals, chronic diseases-causing free radicals, and substances that are harmful to the body cells. It stimulates the body immune system. Selenium is a component of enzyme that activates thyroid hormone. It plays a role in the detoxification processes of the body. And it protects the body against virus invasion namely, HIV (21, 52, 52, 55, 56).

Toxicity

Abnormal level of selenium in the blood called selenosis, which is harmful to the body.

Sources

Plants: Fruits and vegetables: All leaves and green vegetables namely, fluted pumpkin leaves, beta leaves, green, tete kale, collards green and red, garden egg leaves and fruits, *gongronema latifolium* leaves, broccoli, cabbage, and spinach.

Seeds, Nuts, Cereals, and Legumes: chia, flaxseed, sesame, and sunflower seeds; Cashew and Brazil nuts; whole grains, rye, and brown rice; mushrooms; pinto, black eyed and brown, whole-chest bread, and lima beans.

Animal products: Seafood, cooked oysters, fish-cooked tuna; beef, goat and lamb cooked, lean beef, goat, and lamb; cooked skin and leg of chicken and turkey; cooked lean tenderloin of pig, and selenium enriched yeast.

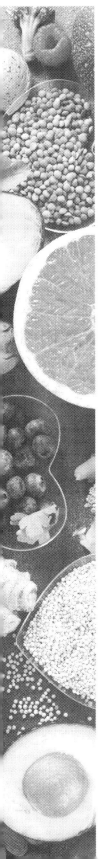

Chapter 38

Micromineral: Silicon (Si)

There is a significance evidence suggesting that silicon is an essential trace element in certain circumstances. Silicon deficiency in rat and chicken caused abnormal metabolism of bone and connective tissues. In chicken it caused abnormal structure of the skull, and abnormal long bones manifested as poor joint formation, abnormal growth of endochondral (within bone and cartilage), low articular cartilage, collagen, water, and hexosamine (52, 53, 55, 56). Evidence also, showed that **rats that consumed diet high in aluminum, low in silicon and calcium, caused aluminium to accumulate in the brain; however, when they were placed on silicon supplement, accumulation of aluminum in the brain was inhibited and controlled**.

Silicon is essential in enzymic activities namely prolylhydroxylase enzyme in the bone tissue culture (52, 53, 55, 56). Silicon is essential in the formation of structures of certain lower organisms namely, diatoms, radiolarians, and sponges. It is found binding to collagen and glycosaminoglycans, as well as in ether and ester derivative of silicic acid called silanonate. It is also found in food additives namely, anti-caking and antifoaming agent. Oral consumption of silicon is not toxic (52, 53, 55, 56).

There has been no negative effect reported on a consumption of an over the counter purchased magnesium triplicate for several decades. Silicon was suggested to have antitheroma (prevention of arterial plaques) properties. Silicon deficiency may contribute to high blood pressure and arteriosclerosis. **It is also, linked to Alzheimer's diseases and ageing-related diseases, and some bone disorders** (52, 53, 55, 56). Silicon is required in preventing some chronic age related diseases.

More studies are needed to provide further evidence to support silicon rich nutrients being linked to affect macromolecules namely, glycosaminoglycan, elastin, and collagen; hence, making it necessary for healthy bones, blood vessels, and brain. Media is yet to pick interest on benefits of silicon to health. Establishment of these benefits needs to occur prior to recommendation of safe daily dietary intake (52, 53, 55, 56).

Based on animal Model studies, rats fed with 35 mg per kilogram of feed and rat treated with 35 mg per kilogram all prevented silicon deficiency symptoms manifested in rat. Silicon is easily available and absorbable; thus, low level may be required for humans approximately, 2-5 mg person per day. Consuming up to 10 mg per person per day can be toxic to the body (52, 53, 55, 56).

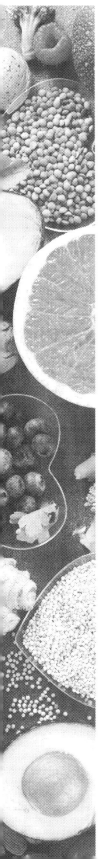

Chapter 39

Micromineral: Zinc (Zn)

Zinc is a mineral as well as a metal, which is required in the body in a tiny quantity. It is called essential mineral because the human body cannot produce it except by eating food that contains it or through the supplement (57, 58). Zinc is located in every body tissue and fluid, constituting 2 g of human body weight. It constitutes about 100-300 ug per gram (30%) of skeletal mass. Only 0.1% of body zinc is located in the blood and it changes rapidly because body PH balance controls its level. About 274 ug/g of zinc is located in the eye choroid, and 300-500mg per litre found in the alkaline are component of the male semen produced by the prostrate gland called prosthetic fluid. (52, 53, 55, 56, 58).

Zinc is needed in small quantity and yet the body needs it for some metabolic processes. Zinc is required for the production of over 300 enzymes and involved in over hundred body metabolic processes. **Zinc promotes good sleep and good health** (52, 53, 55, 56, 57, 58). Zinc **stabilizes membranes and cell structure, thus, giving strength to the organs and cells**. Zinc is essential in a kind of **gene expression** called polynucleotide transcription making it essential to all forms of life.

Zinc is found in all parts of the body namely, organs, tissues, bones, fluids, and the body cells. About 90% of the human body zinc is located in the muscle, and bones. It promotes **cell division and growth**. It enhances the **male fertility including the testosterone** level (52, 53, 55, 56, 57, 58, 59). Zinc plays a key role at **boosting the immunity** of the body, **increases the senses such as the sight, taste, smell and appetite**. Good for the skin, hair and nails. All demography of humans need zinc namely, babies, infants, children, and adolescents. Youth, adult, pregnant women, and nursing mothers, and the seniors all need zinc (51, 52, 53, 55, 58). Taking 4-8 grams of zinc results in toxicity. **High zinc dose of 450 mg - 660 mg per day can lower copper and iron levels**, which also affects the body immunity negatively because, copper and iron plays a major role in boosting body immunity. Upper limit of zinc intake for adult is 45 mg per day, and 23-28 mg per day for children.

Zinc boosts the body immune system, 50mg per day is highly beneficial to health. When zinc gets into the human cells it can prevent any microbe such as virus, fungi and bacteria or a disease-causing organism including covid-19 from thriving. Including zinc into the first aid box will be beneficial (52, 53, 55, 56).

Metabolism and Homeostasis

Zinc metabolism and homeostasis is all about how zinc gets into the body, and out of the body, as well as maintaining optimum zinc balance in the body. It is usually encouraged that organic sources of nutrient are more beneficial to the body but in the case of zinc, consuming aqueous solution of zinc is more easily available and absorbable to the body than zinc obtained from solid food. Zinc is located throughout the intestine. The more you consume zinc the higher it is lost. Zinc can be lost through the urine, sweat, intestine, and epithelial cells. Absorption of zinc from solid diet is less efficient than liquid. About 0.5 mg - 3mg per day is lost through the intestine. Through the urine and integument cells, 0.5 mg - 0.7 mg is lost daily by each. The human body cannot store zinc, although zinc's involvement in over 300 enzymic metabolic activities make it seem as if it is stored in the body (49, 50, 51, 53).

Zinc can be reused for metabolic activities. Up to 2.6 - 3.6 mg of zinc from dietary form can support normal enzyme containing zinc activities for several months. Severe deficiency of zinc results into low zinc levels in the blood, hair, blood cells, plasma, and low urine excretion of zinc (51, 52, 53, 55). The effect of zinc deficiency first manifests in low immunity, prior to depletion of zinc concentration in the plasma. Lactating mothers milk contains 2-3 mg per litre in the first month, 1.4 mg per litre in the next two-three months, and drops to 0.9 mg per litre after three months. You can see that lactating mothers loss significant amount of their blood zinc through breast feeding. That explains the **essentiality of mother's first breast milk called colostrum for baby's good health. It boost the baby's immunity and protects the baby from diseases** invasion.

Recommended Daily Allowance (RDA) of Zinc

Pregnant women aged 14 and 18 need:13 mg per day.

Pregnant women aged 19 and older need 11 mg per day.

Lactating mothers aged 14 and 18 require 14 mg per day, and Lactating mothers 19 and older require 12 mg daily.

Infants less than six months old: 120 and 140 ug per kilogram weight of baby girl and boy respectively per day.

Infants aged six-12 months: 33 ug per day

Children 1-10 years: 30 ug per gram

Adolescents: 23 ug per gram

Male adolescent at puberty: 0.5 mg per day

Women 19 and older require 8 mg per day.

Male from 14 and above require 11 mg per day.

Elderly: Experience low zinc concentration and therefore, they require more than other adults (51, 52, 53, 55, 58).

Food Sources

Plant Sources: Zinc occurs in Fruits and vegetables, fluted pumpkin leaves, green tete, bitter leaves, garden egg leaves, and fruits, kale, collards green, or red, spinach, squash seeds, nuts-cashew, leavened or yeast fermented whole grain cereals, toasted wheat germ, beans example cooked chickpeas, and cooked white mushrooms. It also found in ginger, and garlic, nuts, and whole-grain cereals. Mother's first 1-4 months breast milk. **Animals**: lean red meat, poultry, seafood, fish, and dairy products (49, 56.).

Functions and Health Benefits

Zinc is a component of many enzymes. It is essential for the production of proteins and genetic materials such as polynucleotide transcription. Its primary function is for organoleptic functions namely smell and taste perception, healing of wounds, production of sperm, healthy fetus development in mother's womb. It is necessary for growth, immune system boosting, and sexual maturation (51, 52, 53, 55).

When zinc is consumed at optimum quantity, it offers the following benefits to the body:

- Zinc is used for treatments of zinc deficiency or prevention of zinc deficiency.
- It is useful for treatment of children diarrhoea and facilitates the healing of a wound or injury (56.).
- It is useful for the human immune system boost, and for the treatment of common cold, and ear infections, and to prevent lower respiratory infections.
- It is good for malaria treatment (51, 52, 53, 55, 58).
- It is useful for the treatment of eye disease called macular degeneration that affects the retina, for the treatment of night blindness, and cataracts (57, 58.)
- It is useful for the treatment of asthma, diabetes, high blood pressure, and Acquired Immune Deficiency Syndrome (AIDS).
- It is useful for the treatment of skin diseases such as: eczema, acne, psoriasis, diaper rash, and dandruff (57, 58.)
- Zinc is used for the treatment of attention deficit-hyperactivity disorder (ADHD), poor taste for food (hypogeusia), ear treatment, and severe injury in the head (57, 58).
- Zinc is good for renewing aging skin, and fast healing of injury or wound internally and externally.
- It is good for colitis ulcer, peptic ulcers.
- Zinc could **aid an anorexia nervosa patient gain weight.**
- Zinc enhances physical activities performance, and strength.
- Zinc is good for male fertility treatment and erection treatment.
- It is good for benign prostrate hyperplasia (BPH) treatment (57, 58).
- It is good for strong bones. It is good for rheumatism, arthritis, and muscle cramps.

- It is good for treating Wilson's disease-excessive storage of copper in body tissues, vital organs especially the liver, and brain; it can cause liver damage and death in extreme situation. Wilson diseases is caused by copper poisoning.
- Zinc is generally good for the repair of the body damaged tissues (57, 58).

Deficiency

Severe deficiency of zinc cause loss of appetite, nausea, diarrhea, irritability, retarded growth, low insulin level, general hair loss, rough, dry, and lesion of skin. It also causes poor organoleptic senses of smell and taste and susceptibility to diseases due to low immunity and zinc deficiency diseases. When **zinc deficiency is moderate, it can result in alcoholism**, chronic kidney failure, malabsorption of digested food. Low zinc can cause **male infertility**, and **major depression** (52, 53, 55, 56, 57, 59). People that consume high amount of alcohol were found to have low blood zinc. It means that anyone struggling with alcohol addiction, who wishes to reduce or quit alcohol may need to determine own blood zinc level with the help of a medical doctor, and if it is low perhaps, increasing person's blood zinc concentration to optimum can help his alcohol cessation program to be successful.

Medium and mild deficiency of zinc cause low growth rate and impaired body immune defence system, poor taste and appetite, and poor wound healing occur as a result of mild zinc deficiency (52, 53, 55, 56).

In severe deficiency, taking RDA four to five (4-5) times daily for six months is recommended and in moderate deficiency, taking RDA two to three (2-3) times daily for six months is recommended.

To treat **depression, use 25 mg of zinc together with anti-depressant** is recommended for **12 weeks.**

To treat **common cold, 4.5 to 24 mg daily**, allow to **dissolve in the mouth.**

To treat **muscle cramp, take 220 mg of zinc sulphate for 12 week**s two times per day (51, 52, 53, 55, 57, 58).

Question 1
Write a short note about zinc metabolism and homeostasis?

Answer 1

Metabolism and Homeostasis

Zinc metabolism and homeostasis is all about how zinc gets into the body, digested, and excreted or lost from the body, as well as maintaining optimum zinc balance in the body. It is usually encouraged that organic sources of nutrients are more beneficial to the body but in the case of zinc, consuming aqueous solution of zinc is more easily available and absorbable to the body than zinc obtained from solid food. Zinc is located throughout the intestine. The more you consume zinc the higher it is lost. Zinc can be lost through the urine, sweat, intestine, and epithelial cells. Absorption of zinc from solid diet is less efficient than liquid. The human body cannot store zinc, although zinc's involvement in over 300 enzymic metabolic activities make it seem as if it is stored in the body.

Zinc can be reused for metabolic activities. Up to 2.6 - 3.6 mg of zinc from dietary form can support normal enzyme containing zinc activities for several months. Severe deficiency of zinc results into low zinc levels in the blood, hair, blood cells, plasma, and low urine excretion of zinc. The effect of zinc deficiency first manifests in low immunity, prior to depletion of zinc concentration in the plasma. Lactating mothers milk contains 2-3 mg per litre in the first month, 1.4 mg per litre in the next two-three months, and drops to 0.9 mg per litre after three months. That explains the essentiality of mother's first breast milk called colostrum for baby's good health, Colostrum boost the baby's immunity and protects the baby from diseases invasion. Breast feeding is recommended for all mothers for 9 to 12 months.

Keeping in thoughts the lesson about zinc next, is about vanadium.

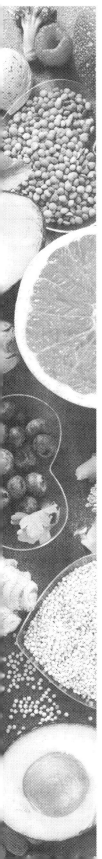

Chapter 40

Micromineral: Vanadium (V)

Vanadium has pharmacological value, and the level required in human is much lower than silicon. Safe daily intake requirement is considered to be 1.0 mg per person per day, or 100 ug or lower may be needed by humans. All elements when up to 100 times higher than nutritional requirement are generally toxic to the body (52, 53, 55, 56).

Food Sources

Fats and oils, beverages, fresh vegetables and fruits contain lower than 5 nanogram (ng) per gram. Next, is about Conditions that affects nutrients availability and absorption.

Next, is about Conditions that affects nutrients availability and absorption.

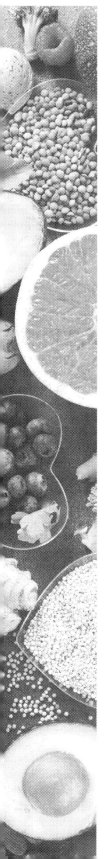

Chapter 41

Conditions That Affects Nutrients Availability and Absorption

The primary regulation or homeostasis of minerals namely Copper, Zinc, Phosphorus, potassium and sodium, take place in the intestine. Phosphorus is absorbed from the top part of the small intestine and is co-transported by transporters such as vitamin D together with sodium to epithelial cells. Copper can be absorbed either rapidly (low-capacity), or gently (high-capacity), and both processes are similar to calcium absorption. Mutation of encoding gene composition of intracellular copper enzyme called Cu-ATpase, which makes the enzyme inactive, causing low copper absorption and resulting in a disease called Menkes disease. High level of zinc and molybdenum from diet can cause loss of copper and copper deficiency.

Food Matrix and Mineral Absorption

Phytates and polyphenols react with metals to cause chelation (bonding), which lowers the absorption of some micro minerals namely, zinc, and iron, and macro minerals example calcium. Phytates and polyphenols occur largely in common crops namely, legumes and cereals. Deficiency of mineral and a significant drop in mineral absorption can cause malnutrition for vegetarians.

When phytate presence is high in the stomach and because the stomach cannot digest it, it forms precipitates of metals and polyphenols, which are insoluble compounds. High consumption of soluble fibres namely, thickening galactomannan gums found in milk formulas, locust bean gum, and methyl pectin can lower in vitro bioavailability and absorption of calcium by up to 12%. Conversely, the use of insulin supplement shows improvement in calcium absorption (7, 8, 51, 52, 53, 55). Higher iron is absorbed in the presence of whey protein (liquid portion of milk) and low iron is absorbed in the presence of casein protein (solid portion of milk). And overheated milk showed better absorption than that of milk processed at ultra high temperature (UHT). Calcium level can drop significantly when there is a reaction between amino acid and reducing sugar called Maillard reaction.

Mineral Bioavailability and Food Processing

Food processing lowers the level, bioavailability and absorption of nutrients and minerals, although minerals resist processing more than vitamins. Moisture, heat, oxygen, temperature affects mineral bioavailability and absorption. And yet, for longer storage, and to prevent harmful microbial activities in the body, lowering moisture and high temperature processing is inevitably necessary (51, 52, 53, 55).

Processing can have positive effects such as making micronutrients accessible through the reduction of anti-nutritive factors. In 21st century, people are having increasing concern about what they get from food such as, good health, liveliness, longevity, and beauty (51, 52, 53, 55).

In food processing, food ingredients are separate from food. After harvest next, is sorting, and coring, then, processing or preparation of the food in food industries and homes respectively. Ingredients are usually added to the processed food before final preservation for safe and longer storage (51, 52, 53, 55).

At all stages of food processing, the stability, and bioavailability of food nutrients and components is under significance threat of loss and unavailability. Minerals resist these threat lot more than vitamins when exposed to light, heat, moisture, oxygen. And zinc, copper, and iron are lost when interacting with carbohydrates, and protein biopolymers (51, 52, 53, 55). During processing, some minerals binding sites are switched or exchanged and this effects mineral bioavailability negatively. Processing involving, heating, soaking, grinding, germination/malting, as well as thermal and non-thermal processing all have impact on bioavailability and stability of minerals. While some food processing have negative impacts, such as high temperature heating, pickling, salting, frying, pressure-cooking and harmful food additives, some have positive impact on mineral stability, bioavailability such as, soaking, cooking, fermentation/malting (51, 52, 53, 55).

Over half of zinc and iron content of brown rice is lost to soaking. Iron, calcium, copper, zinc, and manganese content of fruits and vegetables are reduced during storage. Steaming, microwaving, and frying lowers iodized salt by 20%, 27%, and 27% respectively. Generally, microwaving lowers the loss of iron, calcium, potassium, magnesium, phosphorus, copper, and sodium of foods. Heating significantly lowers vitamin C content of food. Sonication (sound energy or agitation) improve the sodium, potassium, phosphorus, calcium, copper and zinc content of apple juice (51, 52, 53, 55). Various minerals are sensitive to radiation. Microwaving cause a significant loss of selenium. High pressure has no significance effect on milk and soy smoothies. Grilling improves mineral content of catfish. The phytic acid content of yam is lowered by germination, and germination increases bioavailability of minerals. Freezing increases the mineral content of leafy vegetables. Drying denatures the binding of protein caused by Maillard reaction (51, 52, 53, 55).

Canning causes a significant destruction of minerals and nutrients, and boiling reduces the phosphorus content of meat. Baking lowers the zinc, iron, manganese and copper content of flour. Blanching increases the ability of calcium and zinc, hydrogen chloride (HCL) to be extracted from spinach (51, 52, 53, 55).

Processing of foods high in minerals especially those rich in Ca, Mg, Zn, Cu, and iron with bivalence ions example $Ca2+$ usually bond with phytate, fibre, lectin and tannin compounds to make them unavailable for absorption. To prevent bivalent ion minerals listed above from bonding with phytate, to make the nutrients unavailable, foods high in phytate are dephytized first in food processing, to interrupt the process (51, 52, 53, 55).

Additionally, presence of oxalates can lower micro and macro minerals except zinc, and cooking, and soaking of tea, leaves, and cocoa and food high in oxalate to denature oxalate (51, 52, 53, 55).

Biofortification of Minerals

Biofortification is directed at using genetic engineering and transgenic technology to recombine plants DNA, and using foliar application, radiation and chemical improve crop breeding or growing, enrichment and modification of soil composition to realize food crops that are rich in minerals (51, 52, 53).

Since calcium, iodine, selenium, iron, and zinc are essential elements but they are not commonly found in plants, researchers everything possible to fortify (enrich) food with these elements biologically. Examples are, **bio iron fortified rice seedlings**, and **calcium bio fortified carrot** (51, 52 53).

Mineral Fortification of Processed Foods

To meet the needs of poor countries that find it difficult to meet essential minerals in daily staple foods, some essential minerals that are not found commonly in foods namely zinc, iron, calcium and iodine are added directly to processed food to increase access to them and reduce the minerals' deficiencies. Salt is iodized to increase access to iodine (51, 52, 53, 55).

More calcium in food is beneficial to everyone, babies, children, pregnant and nursing mothers, adults, and seniors. Optimum calcium consumption prevents osteoporosis, colon cancer, kidney stone, and hypertension (51, 52, 53, 55).

Zinc fortification is necessary because, its deficiency results in low appetite, and poor taste, weak immunity, delayed wound healing. An example of fortified zinc is zinc phosphate. Zinc Phosphate is better than zinc oxide, zinc chloride, and zinc citrate. Also, deficiency of zinc causes skin and eye lesions, hair loss, delayed sexual maturation, weight loss, impotency, and extreme deficiency of zinc can cause mental lethargy (51, 52, 53, 55).

Iodine is a caritas element for producing thyroid hormone, and its deficiency, lack, and poor use of iodine can cause goiter disorder or enlargement of thyroid gland, and thyroid gland is a critical hormone that is involved in all major biochemical and metabolic processes in the body. It is essential for development, growth, and reproduction. Iodine deficiency causes infertility, Salt is iodized to make it available to all both rich and poor. In United States, the federal recommended dietary allowance (FDA) for iodine salt fortification ranges from 45-76 mg iodine per kilogram of salt (51, 52, 53, 55).

Some foods are fortified with sodium selenate and sodium selenite to increase access and availability. Deficiency of selenium cause hair loss, discolouration of fingernails and skin, fatigue, foggy head, anxiety, poor concentration, and depression, hypothyroidism, and reproductive problems for men and women (51, 52, 53, 55).

Fortification some times masks the original taste of fortified foods, to cause taste inhibition, or masking, encapsulation process is adopted. During storage, significant amount of fortified minerals are lost. Example of such are parboiled milled rice fortified with potassium iodide (KI), and basmati rice grain fortified with ferric sodium ethylenediaminetetraacetate (NaFeEDTA), and ferrous sulphate (FeSo4) (51, 52, 53, 55).

With the lesson about the conditions that affect nutrients availability and absorption, next, is more lesson about water.

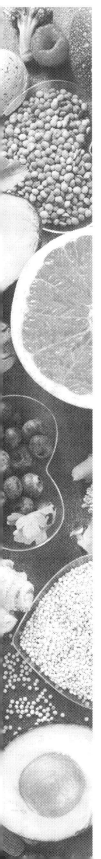

Chapter 42

Water- H_2O

Water is vital to every living thing, human, animal, and plant alike. Water is an essential part of a balanced diet (65). It is made of hydrogen and oxygen, two parts of hydrogen (H + H), and one part of oxygen (O). It is believed that water is life, and there is a common saying that acknowledges that life begins in water. This remains a fact till today. Before creation, the earth surface was covered with water only. In the formation of every animal, such as in reproduction, the spermatozoa and the egg that mixes up to form foetus (young in the mother's womb) come in the form of liquid substance. It remains liquid or semi-liquid in its early formation stage, and firms up as the baby matures. The human body is made up of more than two-third (2/3) proportion of water (5, 10, 65).

Approximately, 85% of the human brain is water; 80% of human blood is water, and 70% of human muscle is water". Water aids the movement of nutrients in and out of the body. All the metabolic (biochemical) processes that take place in the body may be difficult without water; such as digestion, absorption, food and blood circulation and excretion of waste products out of the body. It also functions as a radiator inside the body regulating the body temperature (65).

Despite all these facts and functions of water to the

body, some healthcare professionals barely consider water as a necessary professional advise to patients in a randomized controlled study conducted in Greece that involved six major countries across Europe, namely Germany, France, UK, Spain, Italy, and Greece involving a total 1980 participants, 600 General Practitioners, nurse 300, Pharmacists, 550, Nutritionist, 265, and dieticians, 265 (10, 65). They know the importance of water and yet, not all healthcare practitioner give water advice to patients. Healthcare practitioners from France, Spain, Italy, and Greece give water advice to patients but those from UK and Germany do not factor in the importance of water consumption in their practice. Some do not evaluate patients' hydration level regularly, and over 50% of Physicians do not recognize the importance of hydration to good health and they do not advise patients to consume sufficient amount of water daily (10, 65). Optimum water consumption is an essential nutrient for good mental, physiological, physical and general health (10, 11, 12, 65).

Environment or climatic condition also affect the amount of water an individual requires in a day. For those living in tropical countries and during high temperature that effects the quantity of water consumed by a person daily, in France the recommended daily water allowance is 2.6 litres per day for healthy adult (66). This is in line with the water consumption experimental research finding of Ahajumobi, Operaocha, Eteike, & Sanni (In Press) that showed that 2000 ml of water per person per daily is good for healthy bowel movement.

Functions of Water to the Body

Since more than 2/3 of the total body composition is water, a large volume of water is needed in the body to avoid body dehydration (5, 10, 65). There are many functions of water to the body; here are some of them:

Joint Lubrication and temperature Balance: Water lubricates the joints to prevent it from rubbing and to absorb body shocks. It improves metabolic activities and regulates the body temperature (5, 10, 65).

Bowel Movement: Water is essential for bowel movement and prevent constipation, and it aids in bowel cleansing.

Kidney Function: It aids in the urinary waste removal, kidney function and health. Optimum water intake increases the efficiency of the kidney (5, 10, 65).

Nutrients Absorption: Water aids water-soluble mineral absorption and it absorbs the body shock (5, 10, 65).

Immune System Boost: It boost immune because 92% of the blood plasma is water, it is essential for blood plasma, which constitute the body immune system. The immune system fluid (water) known as lymphatic fluid helps to cure and prevent diseases from entering the body (5, 10, 65).

Energy Release: It aids the expulsion of water and energy out of the body hence; it increases weight loss.

Eye Health: Water is good for your eyes and vision.

Skin Health: Water promotes the turbidity and renewal of the skin and muscles. Habitual regular optimum water consumption moisturizes the skin and delays aging (anti-aging).Washing the face in the morning and evening with room temperature water revitalizes and renews the facial skin (5).

Deficiency

Dehydration or shortage of water in the body affect human health and well being as well as performance. Dehydration is part of of the foundational causes of metabolic syndrome diseases. Up to one to four percent (1% to 4%) loss of fluid can cause poor athletic performance. Low hydration affects appetite and body temperature regulation negatively, and it affects motor control and cognitive function essentially, when water shortage results from exercise performed when the temperature is too high. Additionally, severe dehydration affects vision, sleep, psychomotor, mood, concentration, body temperature and breathing rate negatively (5, 10, 65).

Constipation, low blood pressure, dry lips, dry skin, dry eyes, fatigue (tiredness), blood clotting, unnecessary wrinkles, and poor kidney functions can result from dehydration. Low hydration is not good for injuries/wound healing, and it can cause knee, back, and muscle aches (5, 10, 65).

Dehydration causes fuzziness, short-term memory, and difficulty with understanding and a person's ability to solve basic mathematical problems and it results into poor water and oxygen circulation.

Low level of water in the joints cause friction in the joints so, dehydration is not good for arthritis.

Water deficiency promotes water retention in the body and bloating up, making a person to become obese or overweight (5, 10, 65).

Shortage of water in the body causes dizziness and affect vision, and sight negatively. Dehydration increases the body stress level and provokes migraine too; because, during critical body temperature regulation if, there is low level of water in the body, it causes headache and makes migraine severe (5, 10, 65).

Ideal Quantity of Water for an Individual Per Day

The amount of water required for a healthy adult aged 18-60 years is 2000 ml (8 glasses) per day for people in the tropics, high temperature, as well as those in active exercise. (11, 12). European Food Safety Authority (EFSA) (2010) recommends 2.0 litres for women and 2.5 litres for men. To EFSA 80% of body water need is obtained from water consumption, and beverages and 20% obtained from water content of food (65). Holdsworth recommends that healthcare professional take up the education of patients about the need for adequate water consumption and its benefits to human health. Temperature and health conditions also, affects the amount of water a person requires a per day.

Conclusion

It is an established fact that macro and micro nutrients obtainable through dietary or pharmacological means possess the capacity to prevent diseases and restore health. Health can be restored significantly with balanced consumption of macro, and micro nutrients and hydration.

While it is expected that many patients or individuals are likely to consult nutritionists for guidance on the effective use of the nutrients particularly, as it concerns the health benefits or harm claims; it will be necessary if nutrition professionals seize the moment to educate patients appropriately (21, 51).

Thus, it would be beneficial if we, start our health restoration journey with balanced nutrition and hydration, and get medical help as needed, and this statement does not override situations of emergency. Professional and regulated guidance may be required to ensure that the desired health benefits are fully realized with balanced nutrition.

Glossary

A

Absorption and excretion: Hemochromatosis a disease caused by accumulation of excess

'**accessory growth factor**' The first name given to vitamins when they were first discovered.

Absorption and excretion: Hemochromatosis a disease caused by accumulation of excess

'**accessory growth factor**' The first name given to vitamins when they were first discovered.

ADEK: Fat-soluble vitamins namely vitamins A, D, E and K.

Alternative: other options of something.

Anemia: Shortage of red blood cells or hemoglobin to perform its function of oxygen and nutrient distribution to the body cells.

Anti-hemorrhage factor: vitamin K. There are different vitamins of vitamin K, such as K1, K2, and K3.

Anti neuritis: "A-N" or anti-beriberi.

Antioxidant: That which prevents cell oxidation.

Anti-pellagra: "P-P"-pellagra preventive.

Antitheroma: that which prevents artery plaques.

Ataxia: Abnormal and uncoordinated movements.

Ascorbic acid: Vitamin C.

B

Basal metabolic rate (BMR): Amount of energy needed by the body when at rest, which the body requires to perform basic vital functions namely, breathing, maintaining body temperature is called basal metabolic rate (BMR.

Beriberi/anti neuritis (A-N): a diseases caused by lack or deficiency of B-group vitamins.

Bio-unavailability: A situation whereby there is presence of nutrient example, zinc in the body but, the presence of antagonizing agent such as phytate prevents its absorption for body use.

Bioavailability: Nutrients that are freely available for body cell absorption after digestion without hinderance.

Biotin: Vitamin B7. basal metabolic rate (BMR.

Beriberi/anti neuritis (A-N): a diseases caused by lack or deficiency of B-group vitamins.

Bio-unavailability: A situation whereby there is presence of nutrient example, zinc in the body but, the presence of antagonizing agent such as phytate prevents its absorption for body use.

Bioavailability: Nutrients freely available for body cell absorption after digestion.

Biotin: Vitamin B7.

C

Calyces: Protective covering of the kidney.

Celiac Disease (sprue): A disease caused by excessive eating of wheat gluten.

Cerebrospinal fluid: Fluid in the brain and spinal cord.

Chelating: A chelating agent has presence of ligand, causing precipitation or clustering.

Choline: the only vitamin that is required in the body in large amount.

Cholecalciferol: Vitamin D3.

Cobalamin: Vitamin B12.

Collagen: A cell fibre in the human tissue that is located in various parts of the body system namely, in the immune system, bone, cartilage, blood, and nerves. Vitamin C is required to produce it.

Conjunctivitis: Eye dies cause by vitamin A.

Cystitis: Bladder inflammation.

Cytokines: compounds that prevent inflammation in the body example, interleukin(IL)-6.

D

Dermatological Problem: Skin diseases.

D3-cholecalciferol: Obtained from animals.

Dehydrogenation: A process of removing hydrogen from from vitamin D to form a hormone-like substance called steroid.

7-dehydrocholesterol: Vitamin d produce under the skin by sun shine. It is present in intestinal walls and other tissues.

Dehydroretinol: Vitamin A2

Detoxification: Elimination of toxins or harmful substances from the body.

Diverticulosis: A protrusion of the belly caused by the development of small sacs in the large intestine.

E

Endocytosis: A cellular process of transporting substances into the cell. Or a way by which external substances are absorbed into the body.

Enterocyte: Cell of the intestine.

Erythrocytes: Red blood cells.

ESADDIs: Estimated Safe Adequate and Daily Intakes.

Essential Nutrients: Indispensable food or nutrients needed by the body for it to be healthy when present in optimum amount, and cause disease when in short or excess supply to the body.

Ergocalciferol: Vitamin D2, Sunshine vitamin

F

Fat: Solid or saturated oil.

Feaces: Stole, human excreter.

Foetus: Young in the mother's womb.

Ferroportin: This is a transmembrane protein that transports iron from internal cells to external cells. It is an iron or ferritin.

FeSo4: Ferrous sulphate.

Food fortification: Adding nutrients often vitamins and minerals to processed food to make up for lost nutrient during processing and to make it richer.

G

GIS: Gastrointestinal system or digestives system. peptic ulcer.

Glycated haemoglobin (HbA1c): A significant increase in red blood cell. It also affect white blood cell count.

GSHPx: Selenium enzyme called Glutathione peroxidase.

H

Hepatocytes: Active liver cells necessary for metabolism

Hepcidin: tiny peptide that regulates iron in the body**Homeostasis**: Fluid balance in the body**Hemoglobin**: Blood**Hydrocephalous**: Accumulation of CSF in the brain, causing leg and arm pain in children **Hypervitaminosis** (hypertoxicity): A condition caused by excessive intake of vitamins to the extent that it becomes toxic to the body. **Hypocalcemia**: Low calcium in the blood or the plasma. **Hypovitaminosis**: Lack of a particular vitamin in the body for a long time It is called deficiency of vitamins.

HRT: HRT means hormone replacement therapy.

I

Immutable: Never changing.

IQ: Intelligence quotient.

J

Joule: It is a unite of energy. It equals the quantity of energy of work performed when 1 Newton force displaces an object to 1 metre distance in the direction of applied force. Energy derived from food is calculated in joules and kilo calories.

K

KI: Potassium iodide.

Koagulation (K): Coagulation: Vitamin K: It helps blood to clot.

L

Ligand: A molecule that can bind with transition metals to form bond namely, copper, chromium, iron, molybdenum, and manganese.

Lipids: Fats and oil.

M

Macronutrients: Nutrients or food required in the body in large amount for body well being.

Macrophage: Immune system tissue of the phagocyte or immune system antigen that fights or prevents foreign bodies or antigens such as bacteria and disease-causing organisms from entering the body.

Maillard reaction: A reaction between amino acid and reducing sugar causing a brown colour formation. Example can be seen after peeling potatoes, within a short time the white or cream colour turns to brown.

Malnutrition: Shortage of major nutrients in the body, which results into many diseases, especially in children. Example is Kwashiorkor, which is caused by deficiency of protein. It affects children most.

Melaquinone: Vitamin K2.

Metabolites: Vitamin D produced in the liver example, 25-hydroxyvitamin D3 (25-OHD3).

Metabolism: A process of converting nutrients or food together with oxygen into energy needed in the body for various functions.

Menadione: Vitamin K3.

Microcytic anemia: Presence small red blood cells in a peripheral smear of blood caused by lack or deficiency of iron.

Micromineral: It is simply a trace element.

Micronutrients: Nutrients and food needed in the body in small amount examples, vitamins and minerals.

MTHFR: This is a genetic variant that prevents a person from digesting folate.

Myalgia- Muscle pain or ache.

Myocardial infarction: It is heart attack. A sudden cutting off of blood flow to the heart muscle and causing tissue damage.

Myoglobin: A protein that binds iron and oxygen in the cardiac and skeletal muscle tissues of vertebrate animals and mammals.

N

NaFeEDTA: Ferric sodium ethylenediaminetetraacetate.

Niacin: Vitamin B3.

Nephrosis: Degeneration of kidney tubules.

Nephrocalcinosis- high calcium deposition in kidney caused by high phosphorus concentration.

O

"ol" An indication of presence of alcohol.

Optimum: Average amount of nutrient needed for the body to be healthy and perform its various functions.

Over irradiation: Excessive exposure to radiation heat that comes from sun, x-rays and other sources that cause the destruction of vitamin D.

Oxidative Stress: cell oxidation, which is the presence of free radicals in body that are harmful to body cells, proteins, and even DNA, the end is development of all kinds of chronic diseases, including weak or low insulin secretion. When advanced it results into gut leakage.

P

Pallegra: A disease caused by the deficiency of vitamin B5.

Pantothenic acid: Vitamin B5.

Pellagra: A diseases caused by lack of vitamin B3 or niacin.

Peptic ulcer: A condition causing the erosion of the duodenum.

Pernicious anemia: An autoimmune disease that destroys gut cells and inhibits B12 absorption. B12 pills cannot fix it, but B12 injection could.

Pherein: To bear.

PKNaCaMgP: Five macro minerals or macro elements namely, potassium, sodium, calcium, magnesium, and phosphorus.

Phylloquinone: Vitamin K1

Polyunsatuated fatty acid: fatty acids with multiple or more than two double bonds that makes fats and oils to be very reactive in the body generating oxidative stress and causing cell oxidation that result in chronic diseases.

Polyps: A non-cancerous growth in the body as well as the intestine. In extreme case, it can be cancerous.

Potency: The power or capacity of food to heal diseases.

Psychomotor: Conscious mental activity movement.

Pyelitis: Inflammation of the mucous membrane of the pelvic and calyces of the kidney.

Pyridoxine or pyridoxal or pyridoxamine: Vitamin B6

Q

Quantity: Amount.

Quality: Standard of something or degree of excellence about a thing.

R

RDA: Recommended daily allowance.

Retinol: Vitamin A1

Rickets: Inability of the bone to mineralize, causing rickets in children and osteomalacia in adult.

Roboflavin: Vitamin B2

Resorption: Death of fetus in mother's womb after organ formation.

S

Significant: Large or major effect or impact.

Sonication: A sound energy or agitation treatment given apple juice to improve the sodium, potassium, phosphorus, calcium, copper and zinc content of it.

Spermatozoa: Mature motile sperm cells or male sex cells.

Spermatozoon: singular word for the plural word spermatozoa.

Synthesized: Produced or manufactured.

T

Thiamin: Vitamin B1

Tocopherol: It is a vitamer of Vitamin E: And it means to bear a child in Greek, which describes vitamin E as a substance that is essential for reproduction for male and female. Another vitamer of vitamin E is called tocotrienol.

Tokos: Childbirth.

Total parenteral nutrition:TPN. TPN is an act of infusing a special form of food usually in liquid form into the body through the vein. It could be called parenteral nutrition.

Tubules: Tiny canals that constitute kidney.

U

Urolithiasis/Renal calculi/Nephrolithiasis: Kidney stones that are caused by deposition of hard minerals and salt inside the kidney.

V

VCE: Vitamins C and E

Vitamers: different forms of a substance or compound example vitamin D2, D3, or alpha- tocopherol, beta-tocopherol, and gamma-tocopherol.

Vitamins: Complex organic substance occurring naturally in plant and animal based foods and in nature required in the body in small amount for the body to be healthy.

Vitamins D2-ergocalciferol: is obtained predominantly from plant.

Vitamin D: vitamin produced in the skin by presence of niacin or vitamin B 3 and sunshine.

W

Whole grain: Grain that is the way nature made it. Containing all its nutrients including the bran.

Whole-wheat bread: Bread made from whole wheat grain flour.

X

Xanthine oxidase: A digestive enzyme that contains molybdenum.

Xerophthalmia: Eye diseases caused by severe shortage of Vitamin A, which is extreme case of conjunctivitis.

X-factor: acronym used by researchers to query substance or vitamins that were then not discovered but, manifests signs of its existence or presence. Examples. X-factor was used when various forms of B-group vitamins, were discovered; when vitamin D was discovered from irradiated cod liver oil that changed its vitamin A to vitamin D. It was also used when vitamin E was separated as a different vitamin from vitamin D.

Y

Yoghort: A product made from milk by a process of curdling in the presence of healthy bacteria to improve the digestive system health. Sometimes fruits are added to it.

Z

Zinc: Inorganic element or metal required in the body in minute quantity.

Zinc fortification: Adding zinc to processed food

Reference

1   Meinhard, James, E. "Chromatography: Aperspective." Science. *American Association for the Advancement of Science*. 1949 October 12.110.2859: 387-392. Accessed on December 15, 2021. Available from https://www.jstor.org/stable/1676188

2   Loosli AR, Requa RK, Ross W, Garrick JG. Injuries in Slow-Pitch Softball. Physiological Sportsmed. 1988 Jul.16.7:110-8. doi: 10.1080/00913847.1988.11709557. PMID: 27403830. Accessed on December 15, 2021. Available from https://pubmed.ncbi.nlm.nih.gov/27403830/

3   McDowell, L. R. Vitamins in Animal Nutrition: Comparative Aspect to Human Nutrition. Academic Press INC. 1250 sixth Avenue, San Diego California 92101. 2012 December 2. 486 pages1-end. Accessed on December 12, 2021. Available from https://books.google.ca/books

4   Sebrell, W. H., & Robert, S. H. The Vitamins (second edition). Academic Press. 1967 xi-xiii. ISBN 9781483197043. Doi: 10.1016/B978-1-4831-9704-3.50006-7. Accessed on December 15, 2021. Available from https://www.sciencedirect.com/book/9781483197043/the-vitamin

5   Ahajumobi, E. Nutrition for chronic diseases prevention and control. 2018 January. Accessed on May 23, 2021. Available from http://www.lulu.com/content/e-book/nutrition-for-chronc-diseases-prevention-and-control/22504853

6   Megumi Tsubota-Utsugi, Eri Imai, Makiki Nakade, Nobuyo Tsuboyama-Kasaoka, Akemi Morita, & Shinkan Tokudome. Dietary reference intake for Japanes - 2010 - *National Institute of health and Nutrition*. Japan 2011-2012 Accessed on December 17, 2021. Available from https://www.bing.com/search?form=MOZLBR&pc=MOZI&q=National+Institute+of+Health+%26+Nutrition%2C+Japan%2C+animal+growth+model+2010, pdf copy.

7   Combs, G. F., & McClung, J. P. The vitamins: Fundamental aspects of nutrition and health. (5th Edition). Academic Press, Elsevier, Inc, London, United Kingdom. 2016 December 15. Ebook ISBN: 9780128029831. Available from https://books.google.ca/books

8   MacDowell, L. R. Vitamins in Animal Nutrition: Comparative aspect to Human Nutrition. Elsevier. Journal of technology and Engineering. 2012 December 2. P 486. ISBN 0323139043, 9780323139045. Accessed on December 19, 2021. Available from https://books.google.ca/books/about/Vitamins_in_Animal_Nutrition.html?id=m0lOQpezjU8C&redir_esc=y

9   Johnson, M. D. (2012). *Human biology: Concepts and current issues* (6ᵗʰ, ed). Glenview IL: Pearson education Inc., as Benjamin Cummings.

10 Ahajumobi, E. Nutritional factors to Mental Illness. International Journal of Advanced Research, 2017 September. 5.9: 460-477. Doi: 10.21474/IJAR01/5350. Accessed on September 22, 201. Available from https://www.semanticscholar.org/paper/NUTRITIONAL-FACTORS-TO-MENTAL-ILLNESS.-Ahajumobi

11 Ahajumobi, E, Oparaocha, E T, Eteike, P, Sanni, F (Completed) Water Intake and Bowel Movement a Quantitative Research study Manuscript awaiting publication

12 Ahajumobi, E, Oparaocha, E T, Eteike, P, Sanni, F (Completed) Impact of water on Bowel Movement a Quantitative Research study Manuscript under review

13 Oladipo, A. Chronic Constipation could be a significant cause if illness. Punch Newspapers, Nigeria. 2019 April 3ʳᵈ. V.i: p-p. Retrieved on May 09, 2021 from https://punchng.com/chronic-constipation-can-be-a-significant-cause-of-illness/

14 Pinto sanchez, Maria, & Bercík, Premysl. Epidemiology and Burden of Chronic Constipation. Canadian Journal of Gastroenterology = Journal Canadien de Gastroenterologie. 2011 October. 25.i: 11B-15B. DO - 10.1155/2011/125491. Accessed on December 15, 2021

15 Akere, A., Oke, T. O., & Otegbayo, J. A.Colonoscopy at a tertiary healthcare facility in Southwest Nigeria: Spectrum of indications and colonic abnormalities. Annals of African Medicine, 2016 Jull-September 15. 3: 109-113. Doi: 10.4103/1596-3519.188889. Accessed on September 22, 2021. Available from https://www.annalsafrmed.org/article.asp?

16 Harvard University. The nutrition source: Vitamins and Minerals. Harvard T.H.Chan. 2021 December 14. Accessed on December 14, 2021. Available from https://www.hsph.harvard.edu/nutritionsource/vitamins/

17 FITDAY. The 3 primary macronutrients and their importance. FITDAY. 2021 December 15.v.i:p p. Accessed on December 15, 2021. Available from https://www.fitday.com/fitness-articles/nutrition/vitamins-minerals/the-3-primary-macronutrients-and-their-importance.html

18 University of Illinois. Protein "Univers" John A. Gerlt University of Illinois. 2014 may 13. Accessed on December 15, 2021. Available from https://

www.bing.com/search?form=MOZLBR&pc=MOZI&q=University+of+Illinois%2C+2014+protein

19 Ball, G. F. M. (2005). Vitamins In Foods: Analysis, bioavailability, and Stability. CRC Press. 2005 November 1. doi:10.1201/9781420026979. Accessed on December 15, 2015. Available from https://books.google.ca/books?

20 Hoeger, W. W. K., Hoeger, S. A., Locke, M. & Lauzon, L. Principles for lab for fitness and wellness, (1ˢᵗ, ed). Thomson Wadsworth Nelson Education United States. 2009.

21 Amagwula, I., O., Awuchi, C. G., Echeta, C. K., Igwe, V. S. (2020). Health benefits of micronutrients (vitamins and minerals) and their associated deficiency diseases: A systematic review. *In ternational Journal of Food Sciences* 3(1), 1-32. Retrieved from https://www.iprjb.org

22 European Food Safety Authority. Tolerable upper intake levels for vitamins and minerals. *Scientific Committee on Food: Scientific panels on dietetic products, Nutrition and Allergies.* 2006 February. Accessed on December 17, 2021. Pdf Available from https://www.bing.com/search?form=MOZLBR&pc=MOZI&q=European+Food+Safety+Authority%2C+2006

23 Institute of Public Health Nutrition Bangladesh. National Strategy on Prevention and Control of Micronutrient deficiencies Bangladesh (1015-2024). 2015 December. Accessed on December 15, 2021. Available from https://www.bing.com/search?form=MOZLBR&pc=MOZI&q=unicef++micronutrient%2C+2015

24 World Health Organization. Dissemination of WHO guidelines and recommendations on micronutrients: policy, practice, and service delivery issues. Report of a Regional Meeting Bangkok. 2014 October 14-16. Accessed on December 19, 2021.Available from https://www.bing.com/search?form=MOZLBR&pc=MOZI&q=World+Health+Organization%2C+micronutrients+2014

25 Donoghue, S. Retinol homeostasis in lads gicen low and high intakes of vitamin A. The British Journal of Nutrition. 1983 October. 10.2: 235-248. Doi: 10.1079/BJN19830093. PubMed. Accessed on December 15, 2021. Available from https://www.researchgate.net/publication16580079_Retinol_homeostasis_in_lambs_given_low_and_high_intakes_of_vitamin_A

26 Norman, A. W., Mitra, M. N., Okamura, W. H. & Wing, R. M. Viamin D: 3-Deoxy-1a-Hydroxyvitamin D₃, biologicaly active analog of 1a-Dihydroxyvitamin D₃. 1975 July, 6.188.4192: 1013-1015. Accessed on December 16, 2021 Available from https://www.science.org/doi/10.1126/science.1145184

27 Nunes, G. L., Robinson, K., Kalynych, A., King, S. B., Sgoutas, D. S., & Berk, B. C. (1997). Vitamins C and E Inhibit O2−Production in the Pig Coronary

Artery. *AHA Journals of Circulation.* 1997 November 18. 96.10: 3593–3601. doi:10.1161/01.cir.96.10.3593. Accessed on December 12, 2021. Available from https://www.ahajournals.org/doi/10.1161/01.CIR.96.10.3593

28   Nazıroğlu, M., Şimşek, M., Şimşek, H., Aydilek, N., Özcan, Z., & Atılgan, R. (2004). The effects of hormone replacement therapy combined with vitamins C and E on antioxidants levels and lipid profiles in postmenopausal women with Type 2 diabetes. *Clinica Chimica Acta,* 2004 June. 344.1-2: 63–71. doi:10.1016/j.cccn.2004.01.031. Accessed on December 12, 2021. Available from https://pubmed.ncbi.nlm.nih.gov/15149872/

29   Holick, M. F. The vitamin D deficiency pandemic and consequences for nonskeletal health: Mechanisms of action. *Journal of Molecular. Aspects of Medicine.* 2008 September 2. 29.6: 361–368. Accessed on December 12, 2021. Available from https://pubmed.ncbi.nlm.nih.gov/18801384/

30   Kale, M. S., Dittmer, K. E., Roe, W. D., & Gartrell, B. D. Interspecies differences in plasma concentrations of 25-hydroxyvitamin D3 and dermal Vitamin D synthesis of kiwi (Apteryx mantelli), tuatara (Sphenodon punctatus), and New Zealand sea lions (Phocarctos hookeri). *Journal of Comparative Physiology B.* 2018 March 28.188.2: 325-331. Doi: 0.1007/s00360-017-1117-2. Accessed on December 12, 2021. Available from https://link.springer.com/article/10.1007/s00360-017-1117-2#citeas

31   Lu, Z., T. C. Chen, A. Zhang, K. S. Persons, N. Kohn, R. Berkowitz, S. Martinello, and M. F. Holick. "An evaluation of vitamin D3 content in fish: Is the vitamin D content adequate to satisfy the dietary requirement for vitamin D?". *The Journal of Steroid Biochemistry and Molecular biology.* 2007 January 30. 103: 642-644. Doi: 10.1016/j.jsbmb.2006.12.010. Accessed on December 12, 2021. Available from https://www.ncbi.nlm.nih.gov/pmc/articles/PMC2698592/

32   Norman, A. W. From vitamin D to hormone D: Fundamentals of the vitamin D endocrinesystem essential for good health. *American Journal of Clinical Nutrition.* 2008 August 1.88.i: 491S–499S. Doi: 10.1093/ajcn/88.2.491S. Accessed on December 22, 2021 Available from https://academic.oup.com/ajcn/article/88/2/491S/4649916

33   DeLuca, H. F. Evolution of our understanding of vitamin D. Wiley online Library. Nutrition review. 22nd Marabou Symposium: The changing faces of vitamin D. 2008 September 25.66.s2: S73-S87. Doi: 10.1111/j.1753.2008.00105.x. Accessed on December 15, 2021. Available from https://onlinelibrary.wiley.com/doi/full/10.1111/j.1753-4887.2008.00105.x

34   Halloran, B. P., Barthell, E. N., & DeLuca, H. F. "Vitamin D metabolism during pregnancy and lactation in the rat." *Proceedings of the National Academy of Sciences of the United States of America* vol. 1979 November.

76.11: 5549-53. doi:10.1073/pnas.76.11.5549. Accessed on December 15, 2021. Available from https://www.ncbi.nlm.nih.gov/pmc/articles/PMC411686/\

35   Chesney R. W., Zimmerman J, Hamstra A, DeLuca H.F., Mazess RB. Vitamin D Metabolite Concentrations in Vitamin D Deficiency: Are Calcitriol Levels Normal? *American Journal of Diseases in Child.* 1981 November.135.11:1025–1028. doi:10.1001/archpedi.1981.02130350029010. Accessed on December 16, 2021. Available from https://jamanetwork.com/journals/jamapediatrics/article-abstract/510191

36   Horst, R. L., & Littledike, E. T. Vitamin Tolerance of Animals: Chapter: 2 Vitamin D. The National Academy Press of Sciences, Engineering, and Medicine. 2021. 500 Fift Street, NW, Washington, DC, 20001. Accessed on December 16, 2021. Available from https://www.nap.edu/read/949/chapter/4

37   Kichura TS, Horst RL, Beitz DC, Littledike ET. Relationships between prepartal dietary calcium and phosphorus, vitamin D metabolism, and parturient paresis in dairy cows. J Nutr. 1982 Mar.112.3:480-487. doi: 10.1093/jn/112.3.480. PMID: 6895912. December 15, 2021. Available from https://pubmed.ncbi.nlm.nih.gov/6895912/

38   Madhok T. C., DeLuca H. F. Characteristics of the rat liver microsomal enzyme system converting cholecalciferol into 25-hydroxycholecalciferol. Evidence for the participation of cytochrome p-450. Biochem J. 1979 Dec 15;184(3):491-9. doi: 10.1042/bj1840491. PMID: 231972; PMCID: PMC1161830. December 16, 2021. Available from https://pubmed.ncbi.nlm.nih.gov/231972/

39   Harvard University. The nutrition source: Thiamine - Vitamin B1. Harvard T.H.Chan. 2021a December 14. Accessed on December 14, 2021. Available from https://www.hsph.harvard.edu/nutritionsource/vitamin-b1/

40   Harvard University. The nutrition source: Riboflavin - Vitamin B2. Harvard T.H.Chan. 2021b December 14. Accessed on December 14, 2021. Available from https://www.hsph.harvard.edu/nutritionsource/riboflavin-vitamin-b2/

41   McDowell, L. R. Vitamin E. Vitamins in Animal and Human Nutrition, 2000b January 1.155–225. doi:10.1002/9780470376911.ch4. Accessed on December 14, 2021. Available from https://onlinelibrary.wiley.com/doi/book/10.1002/9780470376911

42   McDowell, L. R.Vitamin K.Vitamins in Animal and Human Nutrition. Iowa State University Press. 2000c January 1. 227–263. doi:10.1002/9780470376911.ch5. Accessed on December 14, 2021. Available from https://onlinelibrary.wiley.com/doi/book/10.1002/9780470376911

43   McDowell, L. R. Vitamins in Animal and Human Nutrition, Second Edition. Iowa, State University Press. 2000a January 1.91–153. doi:10.1002/9780470376911.ch3. Accessed on December 14, 2021. Available from https://onlinelibrary.wiley.com/doi/book/10.1002/9780470376911

44   McDowell, L. R. Vitamin-Like Substances. Vitamins in Animal and Human Nutrition. Iowa State University. 2000 January 1. 659–674. doi:10.1002/9780470376911.ch17. Accessed on December 14, 2021. Available from https://onlinelibrary.wiley.com/doi/book/doi:10.1002/9780470376911

45   Harvard University. The nutrition source: Niacin - Vitamin B3. Harvard T.H.Chan. 2021c December 14. Accessed on December 14, 2021. Available from https://www.hsph.harvard.edu/nutritionsource/niacin-vitamin-b3

46   Harvard University. The nutrition source: Pantothenic Acid - Vitamin B5. Harvard T.H.Chan. 2021d December 14. Accessed on December 14, 2021. Available from https://www.hsph.harvard.edu/nutritionsource/pantothenic-acid-vitamin-b5/

47   Harvard University. The nutrition source: Pyridoxin - Vitamin B6. Harvard T.H.Chan. 2021e December 14. Accessed on December 14, 2021. Available from https://www.hsph.harvard.edu/nutritionsource/vitamin-b6/

48   Harvard University. The nutrition source: Biotin - Vitamin B7. Harvard T.H.Chan. 2021f December 14. Accessed on December 14, 2021. Available from https://www.hsph.harvard.edu/nutritionsource/biotin-vitamin-b7/

49   Harvard University. The nutrition source: Folate(Folic Acid) - Vitamin B9. Harvard T.H.Chan. 2021g December 14. Accessed on December 14, 2021. Available from https://www.hsph.harvard.edu/nutritionsource/folic-acid/

50   Harvard University. The nutrition source: Vitamin B12. Harvard T.H.Chan. 2021h December 15. Accessed on December 15, 2021. Available from https://www.hsph.harvard.edu/nutritionsource/vitamin-b12/

51   Gharibzahedi, S. M. T., & Jafari, S. M. The importance of minerals in human nutrition: Bioavailability, food fortification, processing effects and nanoencapsulation. *Trends in Food Science & Technology*. 2017 April.62.i:119–132. doi:10.1016/j.tifs.2017.02.017

52   Heizer, W. D. Clinical Nutrition of the Essential Trace Elements and Minerals. The guide for health professionals. Journal of Gastroenterology. 2002 March. 122.3: 834-p. Accessed on December 12, 2021. Available from https://www.sciencedirect.com/science/article/abs/pii/S0016508502801445

53   Bogden J.D. The Essential Trace Elements and Minerals. In: Bogden J.D., Klevay L.M. (eds) Clinical Nutrition of the Essential Trace Elements and Minerals. Nutrition ◊ and ◊ Health. Humana Press, Totowa. 2000 Doi: 10.1007/978-1-59259-040-7_1. Accessed on December 12, 2021. Available from https://link.springer.com/chapter/10.1007/978-1-59259-040-7_1#citeas

54   Bogben, J. D. (2000). Clinical nutrition of the essential trace elements and minerals. Springer Science Business media. New york, U. S. A. 2-end. Retrieved from https://books.google.ca/books

55   Castillo-Durán, C., & Cassorla, F. Trace Minerals in Human Growth and Development. *Journal of Pediatric Endocrinology and Metabolism,* 1999

September 1.12.5: 589-601. doi:10.1515/jpem.1999.12.5.589. Accessed on December 12, 2021. Available from https://www.degruyter.com/document/doi/10.1515/JPEM.1999.12.5.589/html

56   World Health Organization, & Food and Agricultural Organization of the United Nations. (2004). Vitamins and Mineral Requirements in Human Nutrition, (2nd, Ed). Online Google book available from https://books.googleusercontent.com/books/content

57   WebMd.com. Zinc. WebMD. 2021. Accessed on December 17, 2021. Available from https://www.webmd.com/search/search_results/default.aspx?query=zinc

58   Zinc International Association. Zinc: Essential for modern life. Zinc International Association. 2021. Accessed on December 17, 2021. Available from https://www.zinc.org/

59   Heffernan, S.M., Horner K., De Vito, G., Conway G. E. The Role of Mineral and Trace Element Supplementation in Exercise and Athletic Performance: A Systematic Review. Nutrients. 2019 Mar 24;11(3):696. doi: 10.3390/nu11030696. PMID: 30909645; PMCID: PMC6471179. Accessed on December 16, 2021. Available from https://pubmed.ncbi.nlm.nih.gov/30909645/

60   Oregon State University (n.d.). Linus Pauling Institute: Micronutrient information centre: Endothelial dysfunction. n.d. Accessed on October 10, 2021. Available from https://lpi.oregonstate.edu/mic/health-disease/endothelial-dysfunction

61   National Institute of Health. Calcium - health professional. Fact sheet for health professional. National Institute of Health. N.d.a Accessed on December 17, 2021. Available from https://ods.od.nih.gov/factsheets/Calcium-HealthProfessional/

62   National Institute of Health. Vitamin and mineral supplement fact sheets. National Institute of Health. N.d.b Accessed on December 17, 2021. Available from https://ods.od.nih.gov/factsheets/list-VitaminsMinerals/

63   Ghosh AK, Joshi SR. Disorders of calcium, phosphorus and magnesium metabolism. *Journal Association of Physicians India*. 2008 Aug. 56: 613-21. PMID: 19051708. Accessed on December 12, 2021. Available from https://pubmed.ncbi.nlm.nih.gov/19051708/

64   Moe, S. M. Disorders of calcium, phosphorus, and magnesium. National Kidney Foundation. Core Curriculum in Nephrology. 2005 January 01.45.1:213-218. Doi: 10.1053/j.ajkd.2004.10014. Accessed on December 12, 2021. Available from https://www.ajkd.org/article/S0272-6386(04)01448-9/fulltext

65   Holdsworth, J. E. The Importance of human hydration: Perceptions among healthcare professionals across Europe. *Nutrition Bulletin*. 2012 February 10. 37.1: 16-24. Doi: 10.1111/j.1467-3010.2011.01942.x. Acessed

on December 17, 2021. Available from https://onlinelibrary.wiley.com/doi/full/10.1111/j.1467-3010.2011.01942.x

66 McDowell, Lee Russell. "9. Vitamin B6." Semantic Scholar. 2008. doi:10.1002/9780470376911.ch9. Accessed on December 14, 2021. Available from https://onlinelibrary.wiley.com/doi/book/10.1002/9780470376911

67 McDowell, L. R. Thiamin. Vitamins in Animal and Human Nutrition. Iowa State University Press. 2000d January 1. 265–310. doi:10.1002/9780470376911.ch6. Accessed on December 18, 2021. Available from https://onlinelibrary.wiley.com/doi/10.1002/9780470376911.ch6

68 McDowell, L. R. Riboflavin. Vitamins in Animal and Human Nutrition. Iowa State University Press. 2000 January 1. 311–346. doi:10.1002/9780470376911.ch7. Accessed on December 14, 2021. Available from https://onlinelibrary.wiley.com/doi/book/10.1002/9780470376911

69 Cotton, S. C., Roussel, G., Gambling, L., Hayes, H. E., Currie, V. J., & McArdle, H. J. The effect of maternal iron deficiency on zinc and coper metabolism during pregnancy in the rat. British Journal of Nutrition [Internet]. 2019 [Accessed on February 10, 2022]; 121(2): 121-129. Doi: 10.1017/S0007114518003069. Available from https://doi.org/10.1017/S0007114518003069

70 Adebusoye, L. A., Ajayi, I. O., & Ogunniyi, A. O. Nutritional Status of Older Persons Presenting in a Primary Care Clinic in Nigeria. Journal of Nutrition in Gerontology and Geriatrics [Internet]. 2012 [Accessed on September 22, 2021]; 1(1): 71-85 DOI: 10.1080/2155 1197.2012.647560. Available from https://www.semanticscholar.org/paper/Nutritional-Status-of-Older-Persons-Presenting-in-a-Adebusoye-Ajayi

71. Scott Frothingham. What is metabolic rate? healthline.com. [Internet] 2018. Nov, 12[Accessed on March 25, 2022] Available from https://www.healthlinbe.com

72. Garnet health. Basal metabolic rate calculator. [Internet] 2016 Jul 1.[Accessed on March 26, 2022]; Available from https://www.garnethealth.org/news/basal-metabolkic-rate-calculator

73. Shoemaker, S. What is roughage and why is it important to eat it? [Internet] 2019 May 13. [Accessed on March 26, 2022]; Available from https://www.healthline.com/njtrition/roiughage

Printed in the United States
by Baker & Taylor Publisher Services